RUNNING:
The Athlete Within

David Costill, Ph.D.

Scott Trappe, Ph.D.

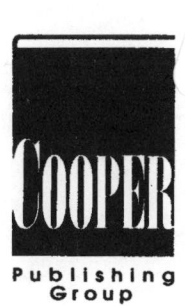

COOPER

Publishing
Group

Library of Congress Cataloging in Publication Data:

Costill, David L., 1936
RUNNING: THE ATHLETE WITHIN

Publisher: I. L. Cooper

Library of Congress Catalog Card Number: 2002105111
ISBN: 1-884125-82-4

Printed in the United States of America by Cooper Publishing Group, LLC, P.O. Box 1129, Traverse City, MI 49685.

10 9 8 7 6 5 4 3 2 1

CONTENTS

PREFACE

Runners and scientists have learned from each other for more than a century. Since the late 1800s runners have subjected themselves to the curiosity of scientists, who have searched for the physiological limits of human endurance. No human subjects were more tolerant or willing to push themselves to exhaustion than these athletes. The list of distance running "human guinea pigs" includes a "Who's Who" of champion runners. Clarence DeMar (seven times winner of the Boston Marathon), Grete Waitz (nine times winner of the New York Marathon), and Emile Zatopeck (winner of the 5,000, 10,000, and Marathon at the 1952 Olympics) are at the top of the list of runners who have been extensively studied in the laboratory.

While the information gained from these and other runners was generally descriptive, early studies provided a physiological sketch of the qualities necessary for success in running. In the 1920s and 30s Harvard University scientists realized that having great endurance demanded a strong and efficient heart, fatigue tolerant muscles, and a body with little excess baggage (i.e., fat). Most runners of that era realized that hard training was essential to achieve their full potential, but little was known regarding the importance of nutrition, dehydration, fluid balance, and the risks of overheating.

The late 1960s saw two developments that had a large impact on the science of running. First, running became popular for health and fitness. Suddenly, individuals who would never have considered an active life after high school became walkers, joggers, and eventually marathon runners. The ranks of those considered distance runners grew from a few participants to hundreds of thousands of men and women. As a result, commercial opportunists were quick to see that exercise could mean big money, and the marketing of sports drinks and running gear began to provide a source of funding for sports science research. The effect over the years has been a rather thorough understanding of the physiology of training, nutrition, gender differences, and aging among distance runners.

Perhaps it is natural that runners will always look for the "magic bullet" that will make them a champion. Some would like to think that "bullet" is in the form of certain diets; others are content to train hard and push their talents to new levels. Often this quest for success leads to misinformation of one kind or another gleaned from other runners or from those with commercially vested interests. Consequently, this book has been written in an effort to present runners and coaches with up-to-date, scientifically based, information regarding the adaptation of men and women to training and the need for proper nutrition and rest. We earnestly hope that this book can be used as a guide for any level of runner or athlete seeking to gain a better understanding of how the body responds to training and competition, nutrition and the environment, aging and other aspects of human physiology.

Dave Costill
Scott Trappe
Muncie, Indiana

Chapter 1
Dissecting Running Potential

INTRODUCTION

In the fall of 1964 the cross-country team was on a bus headed for a college meet when I (D. Costill) got into a heated debate with one of the team's best runners. Are athletes born or made? My debate opponent, a future All-American and National Champion distance runner, was convinced that anyone could become a champion runner, "if they just trained hard enough." I, an aspiring exercise physiologist and team coach, took the position that an athlete must first be genetically gifted and that training would bring out the champion within. I guess my position was not well defended, but fortunately the discussion ended without any punches being thrown. In retrospect, it was just such a debate that led me to spend a great deal of time, energy, and research money on testing distance runners.

Why are some runners so much better than others? Why was I such a mediocre, others might say "poor," runner? Could it be that my 1964 position was correct, and that some individuals are born with "better stuff" than others? At the time of my debate I was attempting to become a distance runner, training as much as 70 miles per week, a difficult task for someone that was a sprint swimmer in college. Although the training had greatly improved my endurance, my race performances were quite average. In an effort to factor-out my limitations, I performed extensive laboratory tests on the college runners I was coaching. Some years later, while at Ball State University, I had the opportunity to study more elite runners including many world and Olympic distance running champions.

In 1966 I took pity on my college cross-country runners and gave up coaching! Still interested in the talents of champion athletes, I began testing as many elite and non-elite runners as I could drag into the Human Performance Laboratory at Ball State University. Initially, I tested the runners, and myself, with every test I felt might influence endurance performance. I suppose it could be said that we went on a "research fishing trip." Soon I realized that only a few tests were needed to separate the physiological talents of elite and non-elite runners.

Over the next 30 years I remained interested in this same question, "what are the requirements for success in sports." Whether we were testing swimmers, cyclists, speed skaters, wrestlers, football or basketball players, our initial studies of each athletic group attempted to dissect the physiological qualities that con-

Historical Note

The first distance runner to be studied by physiologists was Edward Payson Weston, a "pedestrian competitor" in 1871. Austin Flint, a renowned physiologist in the late 1800s, studied Weston's diet and urinary excretion of nitrogen during 5-days of running and walking a total of 317.5 miles.

1

tributed to the athlete's successes or failures. In the remainder of this chapter we'll consider which factors might limit your potential as a runner, some advantages and some handicaps.

BODY SHAPE AND COMPOSITION

Stand at the start of any distance running event and it becomes readily apparent that runners come in all shapes and sizes. If you are still around for the finish of the race, it is equally obvious that the early finishers tend to be alike in at least one respect. They are all lean and thin! As in most sports, physique can work to help or hinder your running form and endurance.

Unlike other athletes who might have greater muscle mass and speed, distance runners generally have little muscle mass, great endurance, and do their best to steer clear of contact sports. Distance runners, for example, may differ in stature, but they all have one common trait — the good ones are skinny. Any weight in the form of fat or muscle that does not contribute to the task of running is, for the most part, excess baggage, which demands the expenditure of energy simply to overcome gravity.

When we first began testing subjects in the late 1960s, we could say with some confidence that on average, the body fat content of normally active, non-athletic, college men and women averaged 14% and 22%, respectively. Students in today's over-nourished and under-exercised society, on the other hand, would be considered thin by those standards. Distance runners, however, continue to be lean. Male runners have repeatedly been reported to have less than 10% body fat. At the 1968 Olympic Marathon trial, the males had an average body fat of 7.5%, a value that might accurately describe the best runners today. Although measured values of less than 4% have been reported for some world class male runners, namely Frank Shorter, Gary Tuttle, and Alberto Salazar, it should be mentioned that measurements of body fat can have a sizeable error and may only be accurate to within 2 or 3% of the runner's "true body fat."

It wasn't until the mid-1970s that there were enough females participating in this sport to provide a reasonable picture of body fatness among successful runners. Elite female distance runners were reported to have body fat contents that ranged from 6 to 18%. In 1980, we observed that the great Norwegian marathoner Grete Waitz had a body fat content of 9%.

Since excessive body fat and bone structure serve as dead weight for the runner, it is easy to understand the advantage held by the runner with small bones and minimal body fat. One might ask the question, "What is the ideal body fat content for optimal distance running performance?" Current research findings do not present a clear answer. However, data obtained from a variety of studies suggest that men and women are in their best running form when their body fat contents are slightly below 10% for men and 15% for women.

For an overweight runner, weight loss often improves performance more than a harder training schedule. As an example, we studied a male runner who weighed 175 pounds (19% fat) and had a best 10-mile performance of 80 min: 20 s. When his body weight was reduced to 165 pounds (14% fat), performance in the 10-mile decreased to 70 min: 50 s. A further reduction in weight to 154 pounds (8%) resulted in a best time of 68 min: 15 s. Measurable improvements in performance can be expected with relatively large reductions in body weight, but it is unlikely that small daily variations of one or two pounds will have any noticeable effect on running. Such increases or decreases are probably related more to changes in the body's water content than to changes in fat weight.

The idea that major weight loss will immediately produce dramatic improvements in performance may oversimplify the situation. There is always the risk that extreme and sudden weight loss will produce some loss of the body's muscle tissue. As a result, sudden weight loss may weaken the runner, drain his or her energy reserves, and result in poorer performances. A few runners may become so obsessed with the idea of having to be skinny to perform that they may become anorexic. It should be realized that fat plays an important role in transporting hormones, providing energy, and structuring the cell membranes. Complete or even partial starvation may initially impair performance. For that reason, it is wise to monitor your percentage of body fat and total body weight at regular intervals.

How accurate are the methods for measuring body fatness? Short of dissecting out all the body fat, there is no absolutely valid method. Since early in the 1900s, the gold standard of body fat measurement used the physical principles of Archimedes, involving the measurement of an individual's weight on land and under water. Since fat is lighter per unit volume than water, it floats. Individuals who have more than their share of body fat have a low density and are good floaters. Unfortunately, this method calculated the density of the whole body and assigned standard values for the density of bone and muscle, assuming that everyone had the same values. Of course, this is not the case. Gender, age, and racial characteristics, all influence bone density. Unfortunately, the most commonly used formulas used to calculate body fat were derived using young individuals of European ancestry, resulting in sizeable errors when estimates were used for other groups.

Since nearly 80% of all fat in the body is stored beneath the skin, skinfold thickness has traditionally been used to approximate one's percent of body fat. Because it is easily administered, this method is often used by some fitness facilities, but is not very precise. In the hands of a trained, experienced tester, this method can be sufficiently accurate to help judge major changes in your body composition. Such body fat measurements should, however, be used only for monitoring your own changes, and not to compare one person to another. Monthly measurements combined with records of body weight can be helpful for runners who want to monitor changes in body fatness and as an indicator of extremely stressful training.

In the past, standard height and weight charts have been used to describe one's "ideal body weight." Unfortunately, these tables are relatively useless for runners since they assume a much higher body fat content than that normally found among trained athletes. The Metropolitan Life Insurance chart states that a 5'11" male who has a "medium frame" should weigh between 150 and 165 pounds. Alberto Salazar, previous holder of the world's best marathon time (2 h:8 min: 18 s), was 5'11", weighing 148 pounds, and had 5.7% body fat (Figure 1-1). From standard tables, we might have considered him to be too thin, but then he was the best runner in the world and probably had an ideal profile.

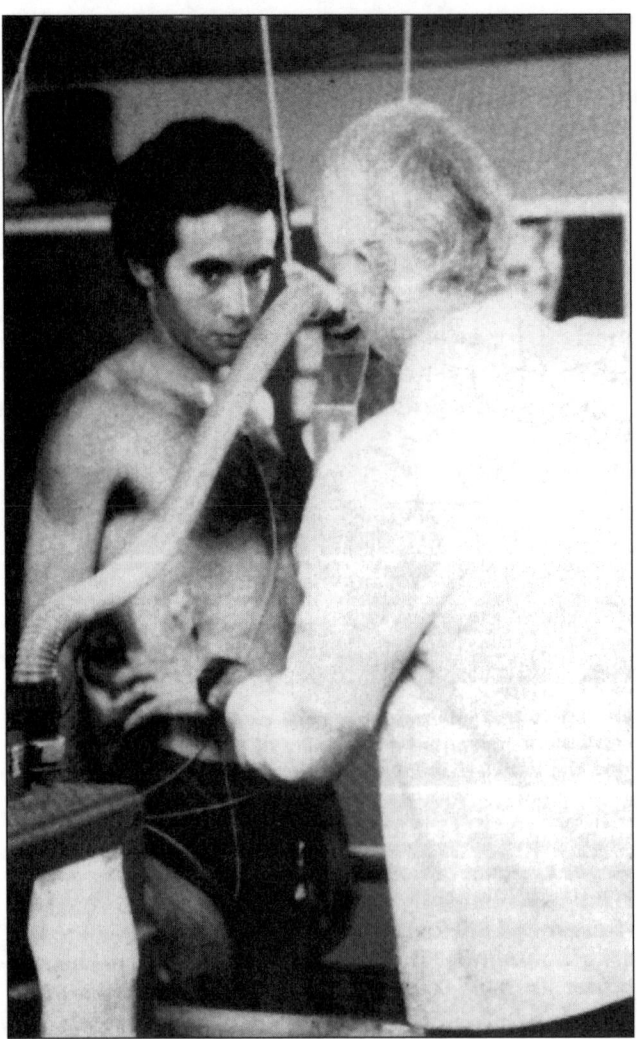

Figure 1-1.
Alberto Salazar
ran 2 h:8 min:18 s
in winning the
1981 New York
Marathon.

As early as 1899, the qualities of height and weight have been recognized as important for successful marathon performance. Early sports scientists suggested that "as the distance increases the runners become smaller." More recent evidence indicates that this is not the case. Whereas the average height for all the Boston Marathon champions from 1897 to 1965 was 5'7", the winners from 1968 to the present have averaged over 6 feet tall. The great Australian marathoner, Derek Clayton, who ran a life-time best of 2 h: 8 min: 33 s, was 6'2" tall (Figure 1-2).

The range in body stature among elite distance runners is wide. In a study of 20 nationally ranked male distance runners, their heights ranged from 5'6" to just over 6 feet tall. Likewise, topflight female runners range in height from 5'1", to 6 feet tall.

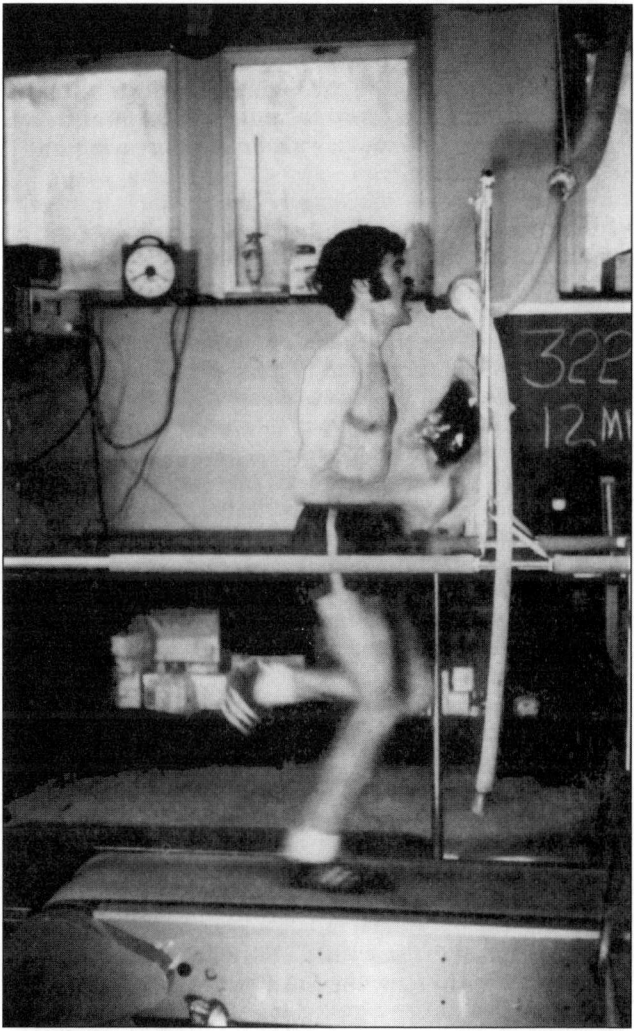

Figure 1-2. Derek Clayton held the fastest time for the marathon (2 h:8 min:33 s) from 1968 until 1981.

Though it can be argued that body type can affect distance running performance, the profile of most outstanding runners may vary considerably. For the most part you can't do much about the body type nature has given you, but what we can say with some certainty is that excess fat will mean slower times. Don't get the impression that excessive dieting or semi-starvation will make you a better runner. Too the contrary, you will see later in this book that optimal nutrition is critical for successful training and competition.

MUSCLES OF THE RUNNER

All human movement, from the blinking of an eye to running a marathon, depends on the shortening ability of muscles. One's running speed and endurance are controlled by the muscles' ability to produce force and energy. Leg muscles are made-up of thousands of individual muscle cells (fibers) that are controlled by a fine network of nerves that carry the electrical impulses from your brain and spinal cord to control and coordinate one's running motion. This nerve and muscle (neuro-muscular) structure and function are among some of the most intricate parts of human physiology. Though the finer points of this interaction are well beyond the scope of this book, you might be interested to know that nature did not deal us all the same neuro-muscular machinery. Genetics, in part, dictate that some individuals are designed for great endurance, whereas others may be more gifted at sprinting. Although your muscles may be more or less programmed for distance running, training can enhance their endurance. Even individuals that have a sprinters muscle type can become distance runners. It is clear, however, that if nature gave you the muscles of a sprinter you'll never be a world contender in the marathon, no matter how hard or long you train.

So, what are the muscle differences between sprinters and distance runners. Thanks to technological advances it is now possible to obtain samples of muscle tissue from runners before, during, and after exercise (Figure 1-3). This has allowed us to study the makeup of the muscle cells and gauge the effects of exercise and training on the nutritional status of muscles. Microscopic and biochemical analyses are used to identify the muscle's machinery for energy production.

One characteristic of muscle that has gained considerable attention from the "world of sport physiology" is muscle fiber type. The following discussion will focus on the types of muscle cells and their relationship to distance running performance.

In the laboratory it is possible to cut slices of muscle samples taken from a biopsy and to stain the cells to identify those fibers that are best suited for strength and power, and those designed for long-term endurance effort. As you can see in Figure 1-4, muscle cells that stain black by this method are the

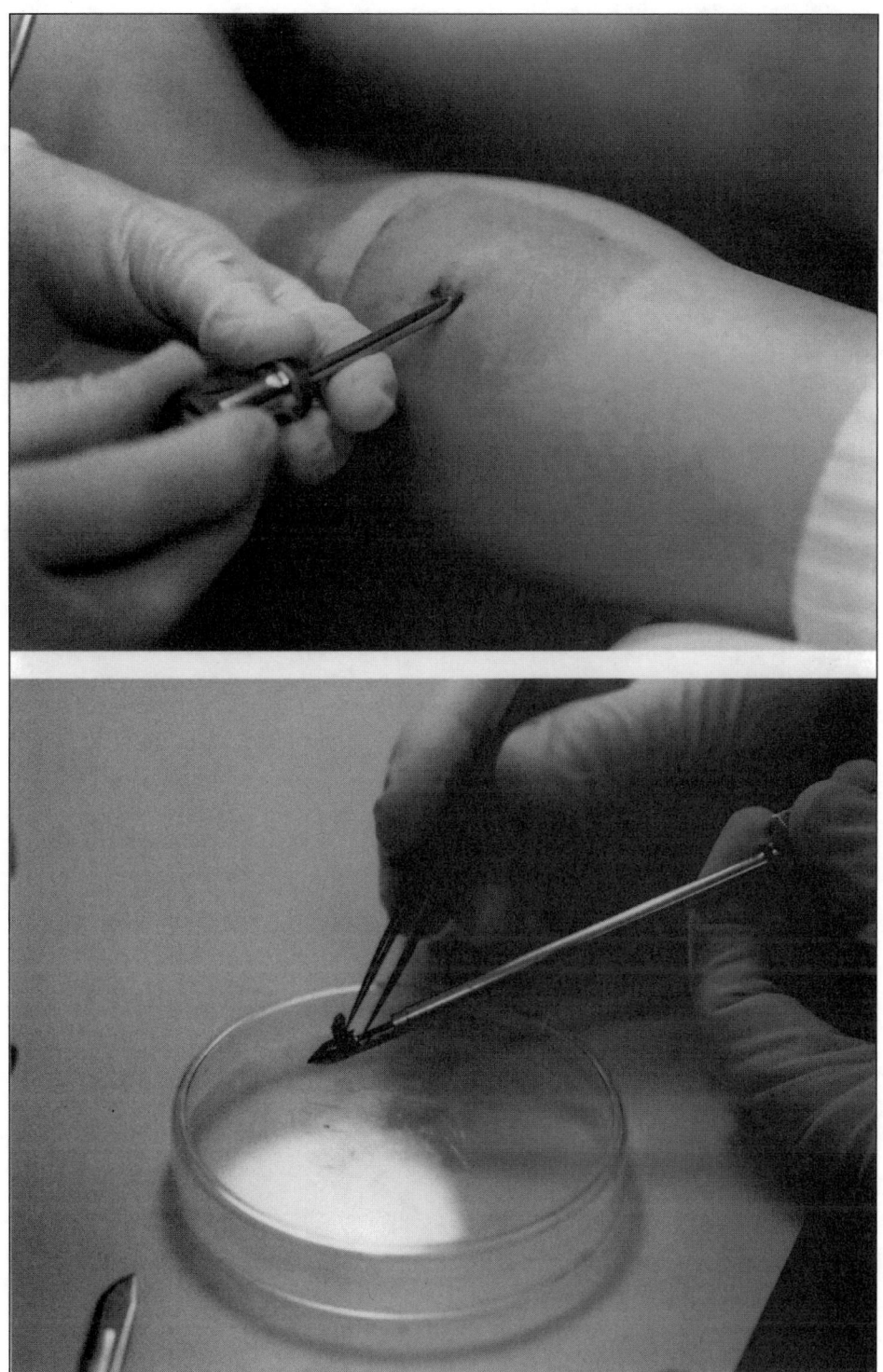

Figure 1-3. The muscle biopsy procedure enables physiologists to examine the composition and nutritional status of runners' muscle fibers.

slow-twitch or type I fibers. Those that appear unstained or gray in appearance are classified as fast-twitch or type II fibers. There are two predominant types of II fibers: fast-twitch type "a" (IIa) and fast-twitch type "b" (IIb).

This whole issue of muscle fiber types can become very confusing, even for trained physiologists, since there appear to be a number of variations of type I and II fibers. All you need to know is that some fibers are good at endurance (type I), while others are designed for speed and power (type II). In the 1970s and 1980s, physiologists debated whether training might cause fibers to change their type. Could endurance training convert a type II (fast-twitch) fiber into a type I? Or, are you stuck with the fiber type you are given at birth? More recent studies seem to suggest that regular activity may cause these fibers to shift their characteristics, but only to a small degree. As we will discuss later in this book, we examined biopsies from elite runners when they were highly trained and again 25 years later, when they were either untrained or only exercising for fitness. When they were younger and competitively fit their leg muscles were composed of 80% type I fibers. Twenty-five years later that percentage had dropped to about 60%, suggesting that with detraining and/or aging their muscle fiber composition had shifted away from the highly endurance type I fibers.

We have seen the same changes in people who are detraining or becoming less active, such as with bed rest, space flight, and aging. For the most part, such

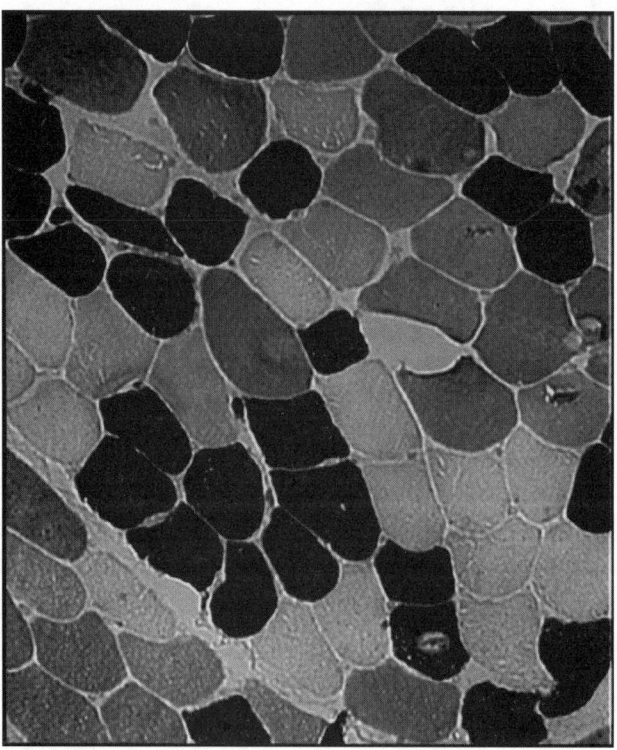

Figure 1-4. *A light microscopic view of muscle fibers. Cross sectional slow-twitch fibers appear stained black, while those with no stain are fast-twitch fibers.*

changes take weeks, months, and even years to become apparent. On the other hand, endurance training may, in some individuals, cause the muscle composition to shift by 5 to 10% in the direction of type I fibers in only a few weeks.

As you might guess, there are a lot of things that can said regarding the changes within the muscle fiber and its nerve supply during periods of training. That might, however, be more than you need or want to know. But, if you are interested in the molecular details that accompany muscle training, we'd suggest you read that material in a textbook on exercise physiology, such as the book by Wilmore & Costill detailed in the Classic and Suggested Readings section at the end of this chapter.

One additional point, however, is that muscle fibers are selectively activated when the nervous system attempts to generate the forces needed for running. This means that if you are walking or running slowly, the most easily activated fibers (type I) are selectively stimulated to contract, while the type II fibers remain relaxed. As the running speed and demand for muscle power increases, type II fibers, those that generate greater force, are turned on adding to the force generated by the type I fibers.

Remember, type I fibers are characterized as having good aerobic endurance and are recruited most often during low-intensity distance running. And, type II fibers create more force, though they fatigue rather easily. Thus, these type II fibers are used during shorter, faster races.

Figure 1-5 attempts to illustrate the relationship between the speed of running and the recruitment of the different fiber types. During slow, easy

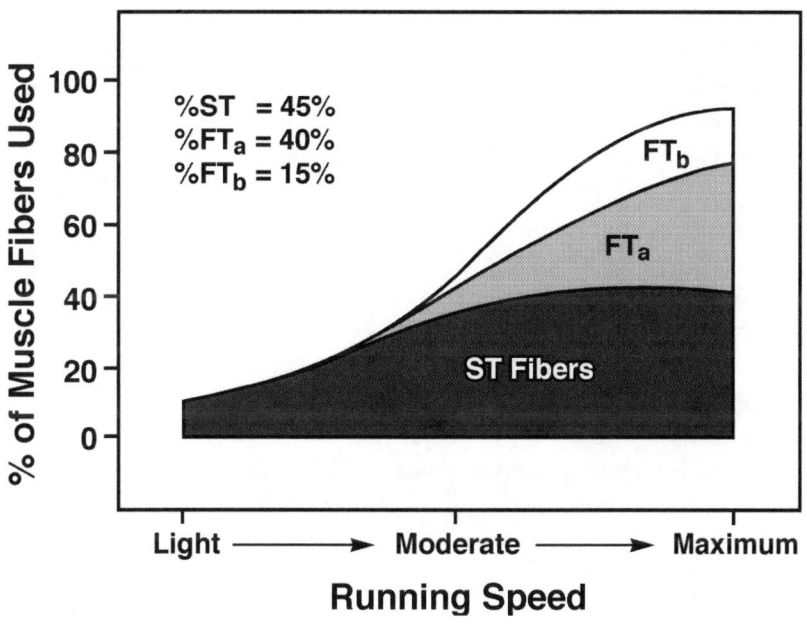

Figure 1-5. Ramp-like recruitment of muscle fibers with varied running speeds. Very slow running and walking may only use the slow-twitch fibers, whereas high speed running or sprinting will require the recruitment of both slow- and fast-twitch fibers.

running most of the muscle force is generated by slow-twitch fibers. As the muscle tension requirements increase at faster speeds, the type II fibers are added to the work force. Finally, at sprinting speeds, where maximal strength is needed, even the laziest fiber, those not often used, are turned-on in an effort to maximize force.

Put another way, running at a slow pace requires the use of the muscle fibers that have the greatest endurance, the type I fibers. As the running pace increases, the nervous system tries to gain greater force by calling on both the type I and type II fibers. However, as fatigue sets in and some fibers fail to respond, more and more type II fibers are activated. This may explain why fatigue seems to come in stages during a race, and why it takes great mental concentration to maintain a given pace near the finish. Much of that mental effort is probably used to activate muscle fibers that are not easily recruited.

So, to be a good distance runner you need to have a lot of type I fibers, and have them endurance trained. Our studies of male and female track athletes show that they have varied muscle fiber compositions, depending on their events speciality. But one thing is certain, elite distance runners consistently have the highest number of type I fibers in their leg muscle than any other group of track athletes. Whereas the average, untrained individual may have a leg muscle composition of 50% type I, 25% type IIa and 25% type IIb fibers, highly trained runners have a predominance of type I fibers. Alberto Salazar's calf muscle, for example, was found to have 93% type I fibers, 7% type IIa fibers, and no type IIb fibers.

At first you might get the impression that muscle fiber type might be a good predictor for identifying potential distance and sprinting champions. In fact, we have often been approached by coaches, parents, and athletes who want to obtain muscle fiber type information to help direct athletes into events that offer the greatest potential for success. Although there is a marked difference in the composition of fibers in the muscles of sprinters and distance runners, fiber composition alone is not a reliable predictor of distance success. The immeasurable factor here is the trainability of the athlete. How much will one's muscle fiber type change with training? How much endurance or strength gains will the athlete experience with training? At this point we are not able to predict how much each individual will adapt to a given training program or which factors are most important for distance running success.

It seems that genetics might be the key to unraveling the mysteries of one's running potential. Studies have shown that identical twins (from the same egg) have identical fiber compositions. Fraternal twins (those from separate eggs) differ in their fiber profiles as well as in other physical characteristics. Muscle composition seems to be established soon after birth during the process of natural development and remains relatively unchanged throughout life, altered only slightly with training.

You might wonder if the composition of muscle fibers is the same in all the muscles of the body. Generally, the muscles of the arms and legs have similar percentages of type I and II fibers, though there are some exceptions. The soleus, a muscle near the bone in the calf area, is commonly more than 90% type I fibers in both trained and untrained people, regardless of age or gender. Someone with a predominance of slow-twitch fibers in his or her thigh or gastrocnemius muscles will likely have a higher percentage of slow-twitch fibers in their arm muscles as well, but, training might alter that ratio.

ENERGY FOR THE LONG HAUL

In order for muscles to continuously produce the forces needed for distance running, they must have a steady supply of energy. The form of energy used for all the muscles' operations is a special chemical compound produced inside the fibers, adenosine triphosphate (ATP). There are three possible sources of ATP: (1) that stored in the muscles, (2) that produced from the oxidative (with oxygen) breakdown of carbohydrates and fats, and (3) that produced without oxygen during the breakdown of sugar stored in the muscle, a process termed glycolysis.

The most readily available source of ATP is that already available for instant use within the fiber. However, this supply is very limited and can only provide enough energy for three-to-five seconds of all-out effort, hardly enough for a distance race.

The energy bound into the ATP molecule is derived from the breakdown of the foods we eat: carbohydrates, fats, and protein. When this process of disassembling fuels is conducted in the presence of oxygen, it is said to be "aerobic." Although the muscle can produce ATP without oxygen, this method is quite inefficient and alone is too limited for exercise lasting more than 20 to 60 seconds. Consequently, aerobic energy production is the primary method of energy production during distance running, which places great demands on the runner's capacity to deliver oxygen to the exercising muscles.

Within the muscles, there are special powerhouse-like structures called mitochondria, which use the foodstuffs and oxygen to produce large amounts of ATP. To speed the rate of energy production and to perform this task efficiently mitochondria employ specialized proteins called enzymes. Since these enzymes are used in aerobic energy production, they are often called oxidative enzymes. Measurement of oxidative enzyme levels are used to indicate the endurance capacity of the muscle and its aerobic potential.

Numerous studies have shown a close relationship between the ability of a muscle to perform prolonged exercise and the amount of oxidative enzymes present. The muscles of elite distance runners, for example, have nearly 3.5 times more oxidative enzymes than those of untrained men and women. Figure 1-6 illustrates that the runner's endurance is, in part, due to the aerobic capacity of his muscles.

Since elite runners possess more type I fibers, which generally have more mitochondria, their muscle aerobic enzymes are unusually high. Even average distance runners, who are highly trained, have large numbers of mitochondria and oxidative enzymes. This illustrates the adaptability of muscle to the stresses of endurance training, even in type II fibers that are inherantly ill designed for aerobic exercise. Even individuals having a small percentage of type I fibers can increase the aerobic capacity of their muscles with endurance training, but it is our general impression that an endurance-trained fast-twitch fiber will not achieve the endurance capacity of a well-trained type I fiber.

ENERGY DEMANDS OF RUNNING

One of the factors responsible for exhaustion during distance running is the rapid depletion of the muscle's sugar stores (i.e. glycogen). Training enables muscles to store more glycogen and also rely more on fat for energy during running. The apparent advantage of performing long runs in training is to improve the muscle's capacity to burn fat, thereby reducing the demands placed on the body's limited carbohydrate supply.

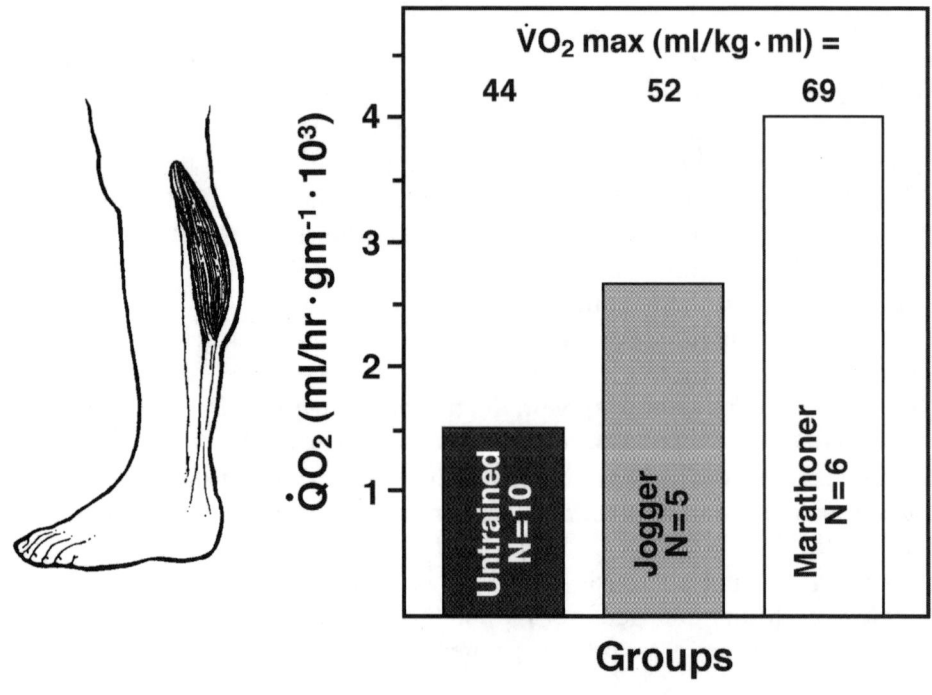

Figure 1-6. Aerobic capacity ($\dot{Q}O_2$) of the gastrocnemius muscle in untrained, moderately trained (joggers), and highly trained (marathon) men. Note that the values somewhat parallel the subjects' state of training. The number of individuals tested is indicated by "N".

The leg muscles are seven times more capable of burning fat after marathon training than untrained muscles. The amount of improvement in the ability of muscles to burn fat depends, for the most part, on the amount of aerobic work (distance running) performed during training. It is essential for the marathoner to perform extremely long runs in training, for only with such work will the muscles develop the mechanisms necessary to use fat as a major fuel. This point provides some justification for doing very long runs every week or two.

Since the 1920s, exercise physiologists have associated the limits of human endurance with the ability to use large volumes of oxygen during exhaustive exercise (Figure 1-7). The oxygen absorbed by the blood as it passes through the lungs matches the amount being used by the muscles. When the energy demands are very high, as during exhaustive running, the muscles attain their highest level of oxygen use.

In the laboratory, we can measure the gases that are breathed by the runner while he or she runs on a motor-driven treadmill (Figure 1-8). In this way, it is possible to determine how much oxygen is being taken from the lungs and delivered to the exercising muscles.

The maximal amount of oxygen that can be consumed by the body is commonly referred to as "$\dot{V}O_2max$," and most exercise physiologists consider it the best single indicator of endurance potential. This point is confirmed by studies

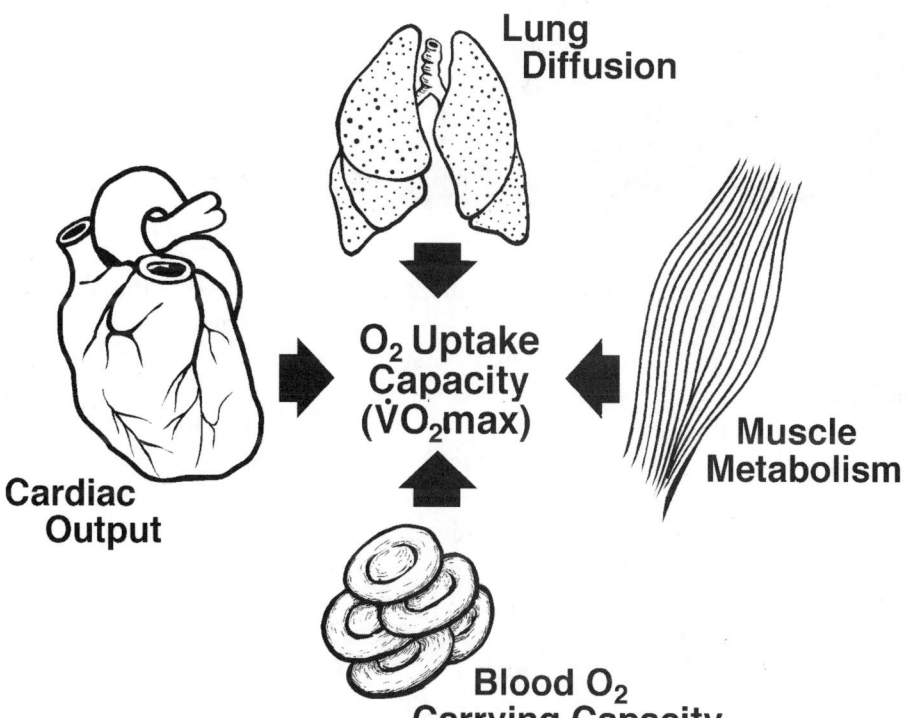

Figure 1-7. *The major factors that determine maximal oxygen uptake ($\dot{V}O_2max$). The two major contributors appear to be the ability of the heart to pump blood (cardiac output) and the muscles' ability to use oxygen and produce energy.*

Lung Diffusion

O$_2$ Uptake Capacity ($\dot{V}O_2max$)

Cardiac Output

Muscle Metabolism

Blood O$_2$ Carrying Capacity

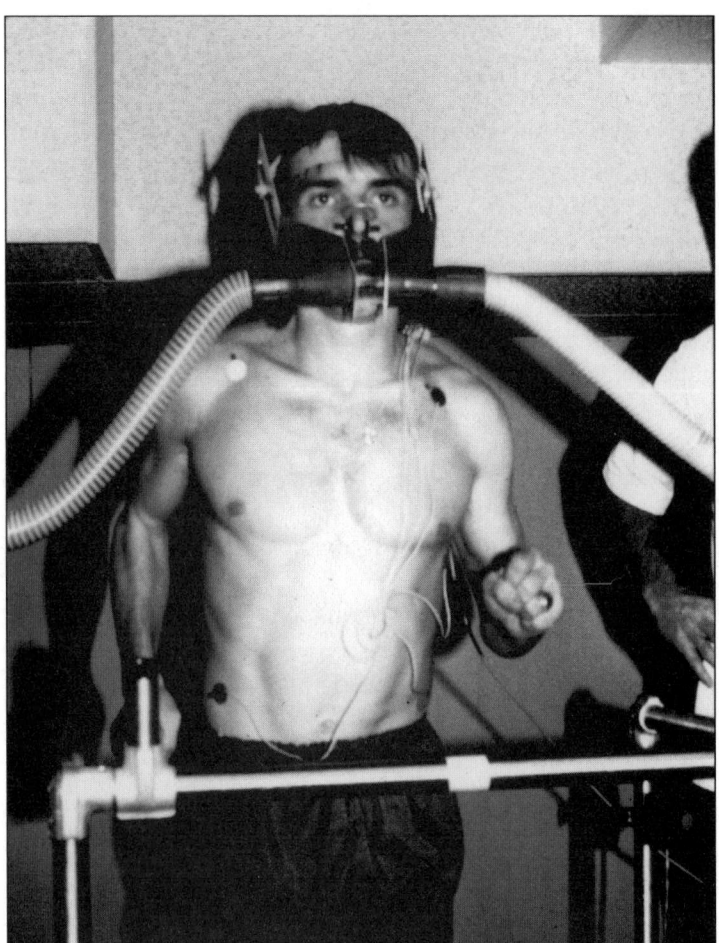

Figure 1-8. *Laboratory testing for oxygen uptake during treadmill running. Runner, Steve Prefontaine, being tested in 1975.*

on distance runners. While the normally active 20-year-old females have $\dot{V}O_2$max values that range from 35 to 40 milliliters of oxygen per kilogram of body weight per minute (ml/kg × min), males are somewhat higher at 44 to 50 ml/kg × min. Highly trained champion distance runners Alberto Salazar and Bill Rodgers, for example, recorded values of 78 ml/kg × min. The late Steve Prefontaine, previous American record holder for the 5,000 meters, recorded a $\dot{V}O_2$max of 84.4 ml/kg × min.

Although this ability to consume, transport, and utilize large volumes of oxygen is critical for distance running success, it frequently fails to predict the winner when a group of similarly talented runners compete. Topflight runners may have similar running performances but markedly different $\dot{V}O_2$max values. This was true in the case of Frank Shorter, 1972 Olympic Marathon Champion, and Steve Prefontaine. Both men had posted times of 12 min: 52 s for three miles. Yet, the highest $\dot{V}O_2$max value recorded for Shorter was only 71.4 ml/kg × min,

13 ml/kg × min lower than for Prefontaine. It is interesting to note, however, that Shorter's value is quite similar to Derek Clayton's, one of history's best marathon performers. Despite Clayton's ability to run at an average speed of 4 min:54 s per mile for the marathon, his $\dot{V}O_2$max was only 70 ml/kg × min. These findings make it clear that a high $\dot{V}O_2$max, in itself, does not automatically make a runner great.

Since it is not inexpensive or technically easy to perform a $\dot{V}O_2$max test, we have developed an equation that can roughly estimate your $\dot{V}O_2$max simply by knowing your best times for different distances. Here are the equations:

$$\dot{V}O_2max = 133.61 - (13.89 \times T1)$$
   where T1 is your time for one mile in minutes
$$\dot{V}O_2max = 128.81 - (5.95 \times T2)$$
   where T2 is your time for two miles in minutes
$$\dot{V}O_2max = 120.62 - (1.59 \times T6)$$
   where T6 is your time for six miles in minutes
$$\dot{V}O_2max = 120.8 - (1.54 \times T0)$$
   where T0 is your time for 10 kilometers in minutes

Example: Convert time for distance from minutes and seconds (5 min:30 s) to total minutes (5.5 minutes). Thus, the $\dot{V}O_2$max based on the mile performance would be:

$$\dot{V}O_2max = 133.61 - (13.89 \times 5.5)$$
$$= 133.61 - 76.40$$
$$= 57.2 \text{ ml/kg} \times \text{min}$$

If you have competitive performances for all of the distances, calculate the respective $\dot{V}O_2$max values and average them. Remember, your ability to perform well during distance running depends on the capacity to produce energy aerobically. Elite runners have aerobic capacities above 65 (female) or 70 (male) ml/kg × min; world class male mile runners are above 80 ml/kg × min.

Table 1-1 will give you a rough estimate of your current potential for distance running success. Of course, this value can be improved with training, so don't be discouraged if your rating is less than you hoped for.

In addition to the aerobic capacity, other factors are instrumental in determining a winning performance. The ability to exercise at an intensity near one's $\dot{V}O_2$max is of equal importance. It is only possible to exercise at 100% of your $\dot{V}O_2$max for about 10 minutes. During longer races, you are forced to slow the pace and, thereby, use less of your $\dot{V}O_2$max. We have learned that some individuals can sustain a pace during the marathon that uses about 70 to 75% of their $\dot{V}O_2$max. Some of the best runners we have tested were able to run at 75 to 85% of $\dot{V}O_2$max during a marathon. Salazar, Rodgers, and Waitz were able to run

TABLE 1-1. Ratings of maximal oxygen uptake (ml/kg × min) for young men and women. The values in the right hand column (Potential 10-km Time) offer an estimate of the runner's maximal oxygen uptake.

Aerobic Capacity	Potential 10-km Time (min:s)
above 70 ml/kg × min	33:00 or faster
65 to 69 ml/kg × min	36:15 to 33:40
60 to 64 ml/kg × min	39:30 to 36:50
55 to 59 ml/kg × min	42:45 to 40:10
50 to 54 ml/kg × min	46:00 to 43:25
45 to 49 ml/kg × min	49:15 to 46:40
40 to 44 ml/kg × min	52:30 to 49:50
below 39 ml/kg × min	53:10 or slower

rather comfortably for up to 30 min at 86 to 90% of their $\dot{V}O_2$max values. So, champion runners might have a higher capacity for tolerating high levels of stress than those of us who run in the middle or back of the pack.

This trait was made clear to us when we studied Derek Clayton in 1970. When asked to run 10 km on the treadmill at a pace that equaled his best marathon pace (4 min: 53 s per mile), he was able to do it with apparent ease, carrying on a conversation with everyone in the laboratory. Nearing the end of the run we asked him if he could continue the run at that pace. He responded by saying, "Yeh, I can run another hour if you want me to." Of course we thought he might be putting on a show for the other runners in the room, so we drew a blood sample from his arm immediately after the run to determine his lactate level, an indication of running effort. To our surprise, his blood lactate level was only 1.8 mmol/liter, a value one might expect to find in someone who had not been exercising. Nevertheless, when we calculated his oxygen use during the run it averaged over 85% of his $\dot{V}O_2$max. There was no doubt, Derek was well within his capacity to run a 2 h: 8 min marathon!

This ability to exercise at a high percentage of one's $\dot{V}O_2$max for long periods without accumulating lactic acid is not fully understood, though it appears that this quality is a function of the muscular adaptations during training.

HEART AND LUNGS

The preceding discussion concerning the aerobic qualities of muscle makes it clear that the key to success in distance running rests on the capacity to deliver oxygen to the muscles. This task is the responsibility of the heart, blood, and vessels that serve as the oxygen transport system.

The amount of blood that can be pumped out of the heart each minute (cardiac output) during exercise determines, in part, the capacity of the muscles to carry on aerobic energy production. It is not surprising that elite distance runners are noted for their efficient, and often enlarged hearts. Highly trained distance runners have frequently been described as having enlarged left ventricles, from which the heart chamber ejects the oxygen-laden blood into the arteries. This hypertrophy of the heart appears to result from endurance training, and it serves to increase the amount of blood that can be pumped from the heart with each contraction.

Studies in the early 1960s examined the function and size of marathon runners' hearts using electrocardiographs (EKG). Though a rather basic way to study the capacity of the heart by today's technology, these investigators noted high voltage from the left ventricle of these runners, indicative of a large heart muscle mass.

These findings of ventricular hypertrophy have been confirmed by x-ray shadow estimates of heart size. Paavo Nurmi, seven-time Olympic distance running champion, was found to have a heart nearly three times larger than normal. We have noted similar x-ray characteristics in our studies of elite distance runners, though not all world class runners show such hypertrophy (Figure 1-9).

The contrast in heart size between untrained and elite distance runners is illustrated by the chest x-ray of Hal Higdon, a world champion veteran runner (2 h: 29 min for a marathon at age 49), and an untrained man of similar age, height, and weight. The lateral dimension of Higdon's heart (15.5 centimeters) is roughly 50% greater than that of the less active man's.

Since the hypertrophied heart of the distance runner ejects more blood than normal with each beat, it is not surprising that the heart will beat much less fre-

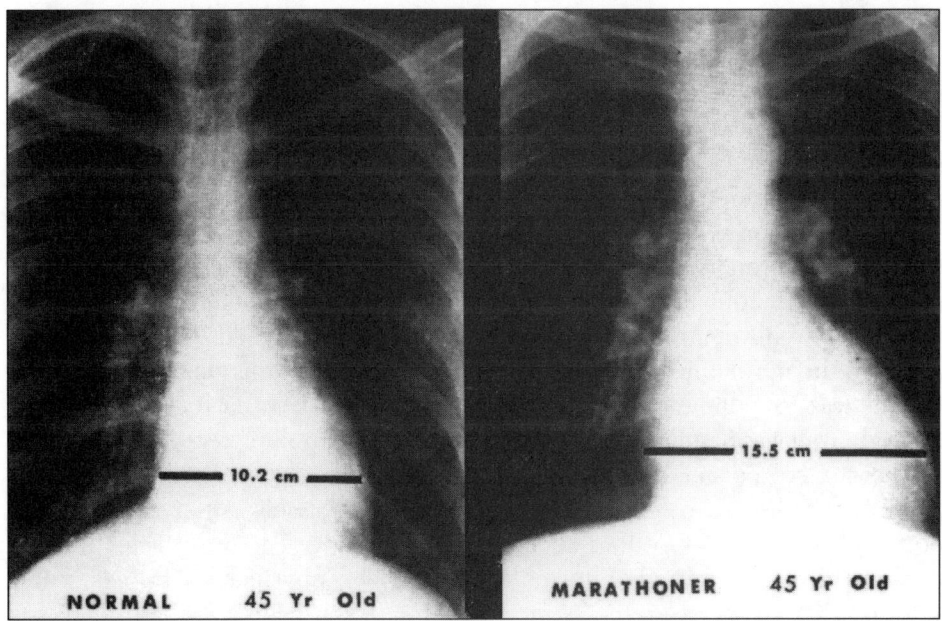

Figure 1-9. Chest x-ray of a world class male marathon runner (Hal Higdon) and a normally active man of similar body size and weight.

quently at rest than that of an untrained individual. In effect, it is as if the runner has a bigger engine that can deliver energy with much less effort. Consequently, the runner's heart accomplishes its work at rest and during exercise with considerably greater efficiency than the heart of an untrained person. Higdon, for example, had a resting heart rate, while standing, of only 32 beats per minute, compared to a rate of 76 to 80 beats per minute in untrained men. If we assume that at rest these men had similar oxygen demands and cardiac outputs, then Higdon's heart must ejected nearly 2.5 times as much blood with each beat as the untrained individual.

ABNORMAL HEART RESPONSES AMONG RUNNERS

A number of elite distance runners that we studied in Dallas in 1974 were found to have a number of EKG abnormalities. Some of these EKG patterns might have been clinically diagnosed as symptomatic of coronary heart disease. Such observations are rare and generally occur in populations that include runners over the age of 40. Though coronary disease might be more likely in this older age group, its presence in the young (21 to 32 yr) Dallas group seems highly unlikely. None of these men had any known cardiovascular disease, nor did they experience any symptoms suggestive of heart disease. Further cardiovascular examinations revealed no additional abnormalities that might indicate impaired coronary blood flow. Although no invasive studies of the coronary arteries were done in these runners, it seems inappropriate to interpret EKG readings for trained distance runners in the same way that one might view that of an untrained older individual. These and other apparently non-functional abnormalities in EKG readings lead us to doubt that such interpretations in exercising, endurance-trained athletes can be of clinical significance.

We have limited access to the results of post-mortem examinations of the hearts of deceased distance runners. However, findings in the case of Clarence DeMar, who competed in more than 1,000 long-distance races and won the Boston Marathon seven times, revealed a significantly enlarged heart with relatively clean coronary arteries (Figure 1-10). DeMar was diagnosed as having peritoneal carcinomatosis (intestinal cancer), but he continued to train to within two weeks of his death. His heart upon examination weighed 340 grams, compared to the normal male heart weight of roughly 300 grams. The left ventricular wall was 18 millimeters thick, (normal thickness is 10 to 12 millimeters), and the right wall was 8 millimeters thick (normal is 3 to 4 millimeters). The valves of his heart were normal, but the diameter of his coronary arteries were two to three times the normal. The very large coronary vessels, other things being equal, would have insured an adequate supply of oxygen to the heart muscle during the most strenuous muscular effort. The physicians who examined

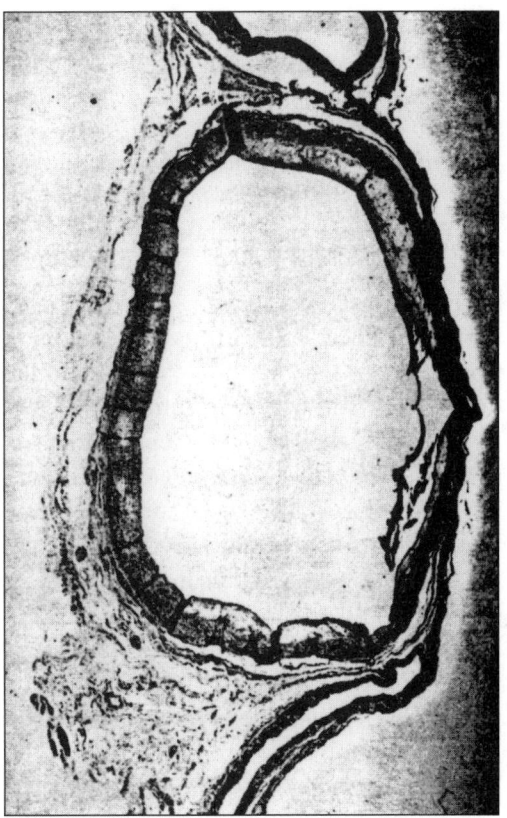

Figure 1-10. *A microscopic photo of Clarence DeMar's aortia, which was 2 to 3 times larger than normal.*

DeMar's heart concluded by stating, "The evidence in DeMar's case, after 49 years of strenuous physical training, was one of notable compensatory change."

Although there is considerable evidence that training for distance running strengthens the heart and improves the efficiency of the cardiovascular system, there is only limited evidence that such activity will reduce or prevent the development of atherosclerosis, a degenerative disease of the coronary arteries. Heart attacks and sudden deaths in older, well-trained distance runners have been reported with increasing frequency in recent years. Though the energy demands on the heart during distance running are great, natural safeguards prevent overstressing it. Only individuals with existing heart disease and/or cardiac abnormalities seem to be at risk during such strenuous exercise.

It is our experience that the frequency of these heart abnormalities are small (less than one in 1,000) in men and women below the age of 35 years. The likelihood of having these problems increases with age. For that reason, it seems prudent for middle aged individuals who embark on a training program of distance running, or for that matter, any intense exercise program, should have a thorough physical exam. Caution should be used, however, in generalizing about the cardiac characteristics of elite distance runners. What may appear abnormal in untrained, sedentary people, might be insignificant in the highly trained runner.

PREDICTING YOUR POTENTIAL

While there are few non-invasive cardiovascular measurements that predict running potential, various circulatory measurements and physical fitness tests have been used with some success. For example, trained cross-country runners score significantly higher than other trained athletes on nearly all tests of aerobic fitness. As one might anticipate, treadmill running time to exhaustion correlates quite highly with distance running success.

Probably the best single circulatory measure for predicting distance running performance is the percentage of maximal heart rate (% HR max) reached during treadmill running at 10 miles per hour (six-minute mile). If you know your maximal heart rate (measured at the end of a four- to five-minute exhaustive run) and your rate while running a six-minute mile, it is possible to predict your potential time in a 10-mile run. If, for example, your maximal heart rate was 200 beats per minute and your six-minute mile heart rate was 180 beats per minute, then your % HR max would be 90 percent (% HR max = 100 × (180/200).

Figure 1-11 demonstrates the relationship between performance in a 10-

Figure 1-11. The relationship between performance in a 10-mile (16.1 km) race and the percentage of the runner's maximal heart rate recorded while running at a six-minute per mile pace. We can predict time in the 10-mile run by drawing a horizontal line across the graph at the 90% level to the point where it intercepts the diagonal line, then drop a perpendicular line from that point to the bottom of the graph. The point at which it intercepts the scale of time for the 10-mile run is your estimated potential for that distance.

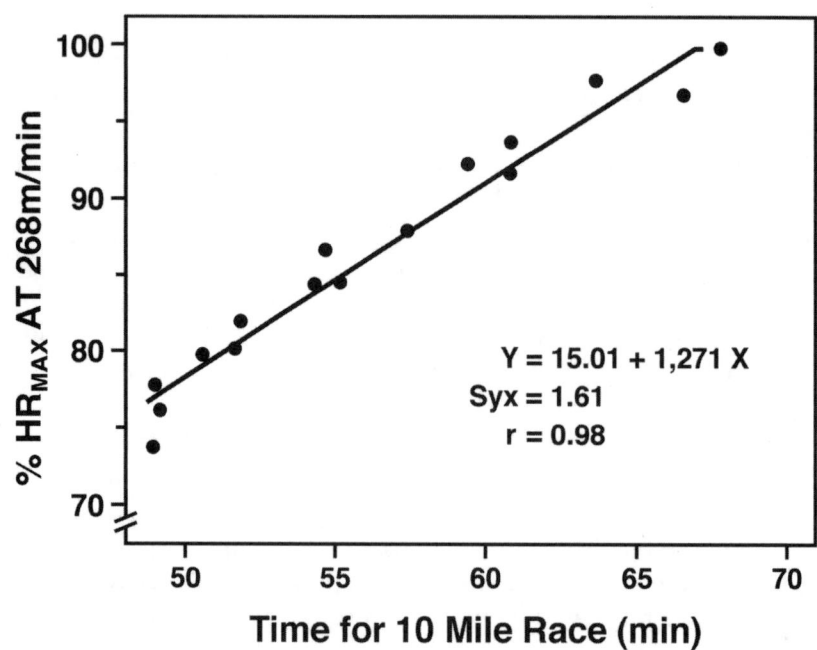

$$Y = 15.01 + 1{,}271\ X$$
$$S_{yx} = 1.61$$
$$r = 0.98$$

mile race and the percentage of the runner's maximal heart rate recorded while running at a six-minute per mile pace (268 meters per minute).

Fine, but what if you can't run a 6 minute mile pace? Well, there really aren't any simple ways to estimate your aerobic capacity, aside from doing a laboratory treadmill test.

In the 1950s some exercise physiologists attempted to show that measurements of blood pressure tracings might be a good estimate of endurance capacity. This concept was based on the fact that when the heart ejects blood into the arteries the pressure is increased. Thus, it was theorized that individuals who had large, strong hearts would have higher systolic (during contraction of the heart) pressures than less fit individuals. This is not the case, however, since training may actually lower your diastolic blood pressure (pressure in the arteries between heart beats) without altering the systolic pressure. Consequently, pulse pressure waves can be very misleading and certainly have no value in predicting distance running potential.

While the capacity of the elite runner's heart to pump blood is markedly greater than that of the untrained individual's, there are fewer, less dramatic differences in the structure and function of the lungs. The maximal volume of air that can be expelled from the lungs in a single breath (vital capacity) depends, to a large extent, on your size. Big people have larger vital capacities than small individuals. Also, years of training appears to increase one's vital capacity. Thus, it is not surprising to find that distance runners have unusually large lung capacities. One study observed vital capacities of 5.7 liters for 17 cross-country runners, compared to the average of 4.8 liters for a group of untrained men of similar age and size.

Training for distance running develops respiratory muscle endurance and strength. Maximum breathing capacity (MBC) is the volume of air that can be forced in and out of the lungs during rapid forceful breathing. While the normal male is said to have an MBC of from 100 to 170 liters per minute (l/min), a group of 10 college cross-country runners were found to average an excess of 200 l/min. One might theorize that well-trained distance runners have developed exceptional endurance in their respiratory muscles and/or reduced the resistance to air movement, enabling them to keep breathing during heavy exercise without respiratory fatigue. Since the respiratory muscles of normally active individuals are generally unaccustomed to long periods of hard breathing, these muscle can become fatigued, leaving the person short of breath and unable to adequately move gases in and out of the lungs.

During exhaustive running, highly trained distance runners have been able to breathe more than 120 to 150 liters per minute for more than 20 minutes, an amount most individuals can only sustain for a few seconds.

While the purpose of breathing is to deliver oxygen to the blood and remove carbon dioxide, these gases must first pass through the lung. Is this process of exchange greater in trained runners than untrained individuals? There is limited information to answer this question, but studies have shown that gases diffuse between the lung and blood more rapidly in trained individuals. Some experts theorize that this capacity for diffusion is facilitated by an increase in total body hemoglobin with training. This might explain, at least in part, the superior oxygen transport system possessed by highly trained distance runners.

DELIVERY SYSTEM FOR MUSCLES

Can a blood sample be used to differentiate between trained and untrained individuals? On first examination, one might be tempted to say no. While there are few differences between elite and good runners, blood from untrained individuals differs only in its capacity to transport oxygen and remove carbon dioxide.

Surprisingly, good and elite distance runners' blood is composed of about 43 to 45% red blood cells (hematocrit), which really isn't different from non-runners. Since the function of these blood cells and the hemoglobin contained within them carry much of the oxygen and carbon dioxide, one might expect the trained runner to have higher values. Though the concentrations of cells and hemoglobin appear unaffected by training, this is misleading. In fact, trained individuals have a blood volume that is markedly enlarged with training. Consequently, the transport system (blood) of the endurance trained individual is greater (i.e. there is more hemoglobin).

Most runners are aware that hemoglobin plays a key role in oxygen transport and are concerned that hard training may cause blood cell destruction and subsequent anemia. While it is true that the ratio of red blood cells to whole blood may be a bit lower than expected in trained distance runners, the concentration of hemoglobin is quite normal: 15.5 to 15.6 grams per 100 milliliters of blood. The number of red blood cells the runners have circulating in their blood vessels is greater than an untrained individual, but so is the volume of fluids (plasma) that suspend these cells. Thus, the ratio (or percentage) of red blood cells to plasma is often quite similar to that of untrained men and women. Though the percentage of blood cells may not appear changed with training, remember, trained runners have more blood cells and plasma, so their total blood volume is considerably larger than normal.

During repeated days of heavy training, plasma volume may increase 15 to 30% as a result of sodium and water retention by the kidneys. There may be occasions, therefore, when the runner's hematocrit may be abnormally low. During the summer months, when training in the heat, we have observed hematocrits below 39% for men and as low as 33% for women. In several of these cases the runners may have hemoglobin values that can make them appear to be anemic. However, after a couple of days of light or no training, their kidneys unload the excess water and their hemoglobin and hematocrits return to normal. Despite these unusually low values, it may be inaccurate to describe the runners as "anemic", since we do not fully understand the influence of such hemodilution on the ability of the blood to carry oxygen during exercise.

Red blood cells are constantly being produced (primarily in the bone marrow and spleen) and destroyed with the production and loss being about equal. There are of course variations in this rate of red cell turnover. Some investigations have reported an increased rate of red cell destruction during heavy exercise, but they agree that this is rather unusual and unlikely to explain the lowering of hemoglobin and hematocrit.

Female runners who experience excessive menstrual flow may become mildly anemic (abnormally low hemoglobin). Though the body's normal mechanism of red cell production should compensate for this red cell loss, there are a number of reports confirming an anemic status in a relatively large percentage of female runners. Serum ferritin, the stored form of iron for hemoglobin formation, has been found to be low in female runners, which has led to a suggestion that they should use iron supplements (see Chapter 5).

OTHER CONSTITUENTS OF BLOOD

Another major function of blood is to transport fuels (sugars, fats, and protein) to the muscles and to remove the waste products of energy production (metabolism). Under resting conditions, the concentrations of fuels and waste in the blood of runners does not differ from those in untrained men and women. The only exception to this point is the alteration in the blood fat (lipid) profile seen in the endurance athlete.

There is reasonably good scientific data indicating that endurance training lowers plasma triglyceride (fat) and total cholesterol values. Some forms of fat are carried in combination with proteins, called lipoproteins. Regular exercise has been shown to initiate a shift in the composition of these lipoproteins toward a greater content of high density lipoprotein cholesterol (HDLC), sometimes referred to as "good cholesterol". Physical training seems to have little effect on plasma cholesterol concentration, though distance runners are generally characterized by a low level of cholesterol. This may be the result of their high metabolic turnover of ingested fuels or simply the fact that they consume foods lower in cholesterol. Nevertheless, a lowering of plasma triglyceride and cholesterol, and an increase in high density lipoprotein cholesterol, have been closely correlated with a lower incidence of heart disease. These changes in the plasma lipid profile suggest a reduction in the risk of heart disease in distance runners. This point has not, however, been clearly elucidated.

Since heavy training tends to alter a number of the items in blood, it is important that the values for various blood items in trained runners be viewed with some caution. One example is the change in serum enzymes, special proteins used by cells to facilitate their internal workings. In a clinical setting, some enzymes are used as indicators of heart and muscle damage. Some muscle membrane damage does occur during endurance running, releasing these enzymes into the blood. Consequently, it is not surprising that these enzymes are in rather high concentrations in the blood following a long, hard run or after several days of intense training. Though the presence of elevated enzymes in blood may be a reasonable indication of very stressful training, the findings should not be viewed with any clinical concern. Some sports physiologists recommend that these enzymes be monitored to determine the runner's status of training stress and overtraining, though there is little evidence to show that they can be used as a reliable gauge to govern ones training regimen.

STRENGTH AND SPEED

On most tests of strength and reaction time, distance runners tend to be below average. Whereas an average group of male college students were found to have a dominant hand grip strength of 117 pounds (53 kilograms), 38 cross-country runners scored only 106.1 pounds (48 kilograms) of force. We might anticipate that the runners would score better in a test of leg strength. Surprisingly, they perform poorly in most such tasks. When tested for vertical jump, the average, untrained individual can jump 21 inches (53 centimeters), compared to a mean jump of 14 inches (34 centimeters) for a group of elite marathon runners.

Although it might seem logical that distance runners, known to have a predominance of slow-twitch fibers in their leg muscles, might inherit this inability to jump, some individual cases suggest that this is not the case. For example, Lou Castagnola, a 2 h:17 min marathoner in 1967, was found to have a vertical jump of only 12 inches (29 centimeters). Following the 1968 U.S. Olympic marathon trial he stopped training and led a rather sedentary life. Three years later we re-examined him and found that while his $\dot{V}O_2$max had declined from 72 ml/kg × min to 48 ml/kg × min, his vertical jump had increased to 20 inches (52 centimeters). Thus, despite a lack of regular physical activity, his explosive leg strength had increased 77%.

These findings suggest that endurance running and the presence of a high percentage of slow-twitch fibers in the leg muscles may impair explosive leg strength, which could have a negative effect on running speed. Recent studies on single muscle fibers suggests that heavy training and/or long endurance exercise may cause some changes inside the fibers that make them respond more slowly and, therefore, reduce the power of the muscle fibers. However, with several weeks of reduced training and/or complete rest, the runners' power and speed are returned. These points will be discussed in greater detail later when we address the issues of optimal training.

DO YOU HAVE THE RIGHT STUFF?

The preceding discussion may have led you to think that the major determinants of distance running success are controlled by genetics, and that you cannot be a topflight runner without the right genetic gifts. To the contrary, the body has an exceptional capacity to improve its endurance with training. The champion distance runners show no unusual talents for endurance exercise when they are untrained. Only with weeks, months, and years of training do they develop the circulatory and muscular qualities necessary to achieve their full potential. Regardless of your inherited capacities, you can be better than you are! The following chapters will give you the facts, as we know them, that will allow you to make the right choices in your efforts to perform your best.

CLASSIC AND SUGGESTED READINGS

Astrand, P.-O. New records in human power. *Nature*, 176:922–923, 1955.

Behnke, A. R. and J. Royce. Body size, shape, and composition of athletes. *J. Sports Med. and Phys. Fit.*, 6-75-78, 1966.

Costill, D. L. Metabolic responses during distance running. *J. Appl. Physiol.*, 28:251–255, 1970.

Costill, D. L. The relationship between selected physiological variables and distance running performance. *J. Sports Med. and Phys. Fit.*, 7:61–66, 1967.

Costill, D. L. and E. L. Fox. Energetics of marathon running. *Med. Sci. Sports*, 7:81–86, 1969.

Costill, D. L. and E. Winrow. Maximal oxygen intake among marathon runners. *Arch. Phys. Med. Rehab.*, 51:317–320, 1970.

Costill, D. L., G. Branam, D. Eddy and K. Sparks. Determinants of marathon running success. *Int. Z. Angew. Physiol.*, 29:249–254, 1971.

Costill, D. L., H. Thomason and E. Roberts. Fractional utilization of the aerobic capacity during distance running. *Med. Sci. Sports*, 5:248–252, 1973.

Costill, D. L., J. Daniels, W. Evans, W. Fink, G. Krahenbuhl and B. Saltin. Skeletal muscle enzymes and fiber composition in male and female track athletes. *J. Appl. Physiol.*, 40:149–154, 1976.

Costill, D. L., P. D. Gollnick, E. D. Jansson, B. Saltin and E. M. Stein. Glycogen depletion pattern in human muscle fibers during distance running. *Acta Physiol. Scand.*, 89:374–383, 1973.

Costill, D. L., W. J. Fink, J. L. Ivy, L. H. Getchell and F. A. Witzmann. Lipid metabolism in skeletal muscle of endurance trained males and females. *J. Appl. Physiol.*, 47:787–791, 1979.

Costill, D. L., W. J. Fink and M. Pollock. Muscle fiber composition and enzyme activities of elit distance runners. *Med. Sci. Sports*, 8:96–100, 1976.

Cureton, T. K. *Physical fitness of champion athletes*. Urbana: University of Illinois Press, 1951.

Dill, D. B. Marathoner DeMar: Physiological Studies. *J. Nat. Cancer Inst.*, 35:185–191,1965.

Foster, C., D. L. Costill, J. T. Daniels and W. J. Fink. Skeletal muscle enzyme activity, fiber composition and $\dot{V}O_2$max in relation to distance running performance. *Europ. J. Appl. Physiol.*, 39:73–80, 1978.

Gibbons, L. W., K. H. Cooper, R. P. Martin and M. L. Pollock. Medical examination and electrocardiographic analysis of elite distance runners. *Ann. N.Y. Acad. Sci.*, 301:283–296, 1977.

J. Appl. Physiol., 34:107–111, 1973.

Gollnick, P. D., R. B. Armstrong, C. W. Saubert, K. Piehl and B. Saltin. Enzyme activity and fiber composition in skeletal muscle of untrained and trained men. *J. Appl.Physiol.*, 33:312–319, 1972.

Hill, A. V. and H Lupton. Muscular exercise, lactic acid and the supply and utilization of oxygen. *Quart. J. Med.*, 16:135–171, 1923.

Hirata, K. Physique and age of Tokyo Olympic champions. *J. Sports Med. and Phys. Fit.*, 6:207–221, 1966.

Komi, P. V. and J. Karlsson. Physical performance, skeletal muscle enzyme activities, and fiber types in monozygous and dizygous twins of both sexes. *Acta. Physiol. Scand.*, Suppl., 462:28, 1979.

Lindsay, J. E. et al. Structural and functional assessments on a champion runner—Peter Snell. *Res. Quart.*, 38:355–365, 1967.

Pollock, M. L. Submaximal and maximal working capacity of elite distahce runners. *Ann. N.Y. Acad. Sci.*, 301:310–322, 1977.

Robinson, S., H. T. Edwards and D. B. Dill. New records in human power. *Sci.*, 85:409–410, 1937.

Wilmore, J. H. and C. H. Brown. Physiological profiles of women distance runners. *Med. Sci. Sports*, 6:178–181, 1974.

Wilmore, J.H. and D.L. Costill. Physiology of sport and exercise: Champaign, IL, Human Kinetics, 2nd edition, 550 p., 1999.

Chapter 2
The Demands of Distance Running

INTRODUCTION

Feats of human endurance have piqued the curiosity of physiologists since at least 1870, when long-distance runner Edward Payson Weston was studied during his efforts to walk 400 miles (644 kilometers) in five consecutive days. Although the rate at which Weston burned energy was relatively low compared to those of competitors in shorter events, the data obtained provided us with an appreciation of man's physiological and psychological limits. The following discussion will show you how the body responds to the stress of exercise and to point-out that the limitations to performance are a matter of energy delivery within the runner's muscles.

NEED FOR ENERGY

All forms of human movement require energy for the activation of muscle contraction (shortening). The amount of energy needed for any effort depends on the amount of force generated by the muscles and the duration over which it is performed. In running terms, the demands for energy depend on the speed and duration of the run. Generally, the runner that produces energy at the highest rates for the longest time is the winner. No, we didn't forget that removing waste products from the muscle is also limiting. But, assuming all things being equal, energy production is the pivotal factor in distance running success. When we say that type I fibers have greater endurance than type II fibers, we are simply stating that type I fibers can more efficiently use oxygen and, therefore, produce more energy. So, having a predominance of type I fibers, as elite runners often do, is a major advantage. Of course, those fibers must be able to receive large amounts of oxygen in order to conduct aerobic energy production, which means that they have a highly developed circulatory system.

The runner's ability to maintain an extremely high rate of energy production for two hours or more was impressively demonstrated by world class marathoner Alberto Salazar, whose 2 h: 8 min marathon (26.2 miles) performance was estimated to cost him 2,700 kilocalories (kcal), about the same as he might have used in 24 hours if he were not exercising. In order to run at such speeds, all distance runners must increase the rate of muscular energy production by more

Historical Note
Probably the most extensively studied distance runner was Clarence DeMar, seven-time winner of the Boston Marathon. He was first studied in 1926 at the Harvard Fatigue Laboratory and continued to participate in research projects throughout his running career. In fact, he even provided scientific information after his death when pathologists examined his heart during autopsy.

than 15 to 20 times the resting level. On the average, distance runners use 95 to 100 kilocalories per mile (kcal/mile), regardless of the speed at which they are running.

That is to say, the total energy required to run a given distance on level ground is constant, regardless of the speed. Only the rate of energy expenditure will differ. When Grete Waitz, previous World Record holder at 10,000 m, ran a mile in eight minutes, she used 35 milliliters of oxygen per minute for each kilogram of her body weight (ml/kg × min), approximately 9 kilocalories per minute (kcal/min), or 71 kcal per mile. At a six minute per mile pace, she would use 47 ml/kg × min, 12 kcal/min, or 72 kcal/mile. In other words, she used nearly the same amount of energy to run a mile, regardless of the pace.

This is not to say that all runners use energy at the same rate or that the cost of running each mile is the same for all runners. A heavier runner would expend more energy because it costs more to carry the added weight. Derek Clayton, for example, weighed 73 kg compared to Waitz's 52 kg. Although Clayton had about the same level of efficiency (per kilogram of body weight), it was more expensive for him to run the mile. Where Waitz might expend only 72 kcal/mile, Clayton was found to use 102 kcal/mile.

THE SKILLED RUNNER

Although most elite distance runners have economical running techniques some are mechanically wasteful, expending more energy than needed to run at a given speed. Differences in running efficiency are illustrated in Figure 2-1, which shows the test results for two middle-aged distance runners, Ted Corbitt (49 years old) and Jim McDonagh (45 years old), who we studied in 1968 and again in 1992. At all running speeds faster than an eight minute mile, McDonagh used significantly less oxygen than Corbitt. Since these men had similar $\dot{V}O_2$max values (64 to 65 ml/kg × min in 1968), one might conclude that McDonagh's use of less energy provided him with a decided advantage during competition.

Since these two men competed on numerous occasions, it is interesting to examine these encounters. We estimated that during marathon races these men ran at paces requiring them to use energy at 85% of their $\dot{V}O_2$max values. Table 2-1 indicates that, on the average, McDonagh's running efficiency gave him a 13-minute advantage in marathon and ultra-marathon races. Since these men had similar $\dot{V}O_2$max volumes but markedly different energy needs during distance running, a large part of McDonagh's advantage in competition can be attributed to his more economical running style. Unfortunately, we have no explanation for the underlying causes of these differences in efficiency, other than running technique.

Various studies with sprint, middle-distance, and distance runners have shown that marathon runners are more efficient than other trained runners. In

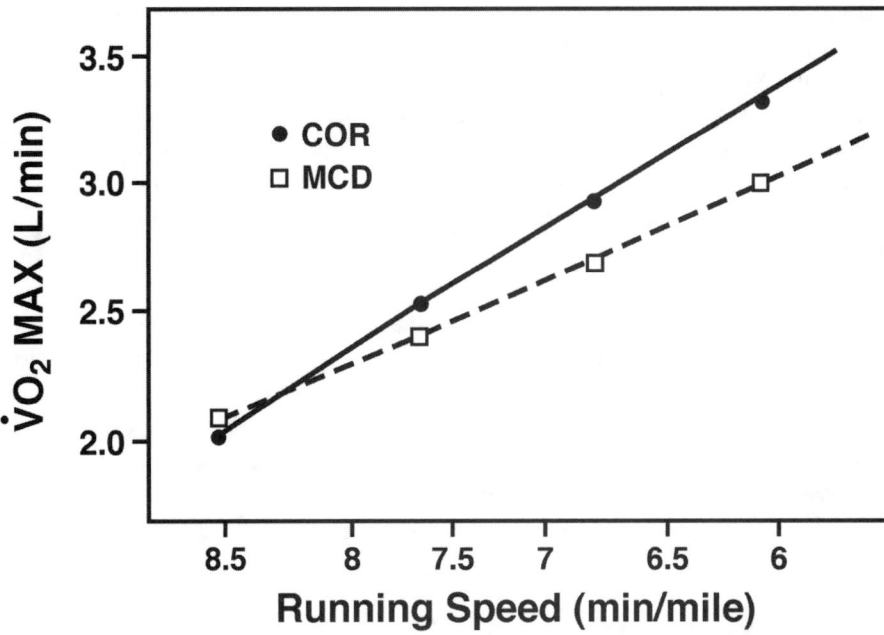

Figure 2-1. Oxygen requirements ($\dot{V}O_2$; ml/kg × min) for McDonagh and Corbitt while running at various speeds. Though they had similar $\dot{V}O_2$max values McDonagh was the more economical and, therefore, the faster runner.

TABLE 2-1. Performance data (h:min:s) for two middle-aged distance runners.

Mon/Yr	Distance	Corbitt	Place	McDonagh	Place
2/67	42.2 km	2:51:40	8	2:46:21	6
4/67	42.2	2:45:20	81	2:29:55	22
5/67	42.2	2:48:08	11	2:30:06	1
5/67	60.4	4:48:08	4	3:36:52	1
6/67	42.2	3:08:42	14	2:43:42	2
2/68	42.2	2:51:33	8	2:44:40	4
4/68	42.2	2:52:00	43	2:39:34	19
5/68	42.2	2:45:37	6	2:36:35	2
5/68	60.4	4:29:17	3	3:50:11	1
6/68	42.2	3:02:54	10	2:46:51	1
8/68	42.2	2:55:01	8	2:36:36	1
2/69	42.2	2:42:40	9	2:37:25	6
4/69	42.2	2:42:02	56	2:29:07	13
5/69	60.4	3:57:01	2	3:48:11	1
5/69	42.2	2:49:41	5	2:39:34	3

general, these long distance runners tend to use 5 to 10% less energy than middle-distance and sprint runners. Since this economy of effort has only been studied at relatively slow speeds of 5 to 10 minutes per mile, it seems reasonable to assume that distance runners are less efficient at sprinting than those runners who train specifically for the short, faster races. Though the difference in energy use between the distance and sprint runners may seem small, it becomes a serious consideration during events lasting several hours. Variations in running form and the specificity of training for sprint and distance running probably account for differences in running economy.

Film analyses reveal that middle-distance and sprint runners have significantly greater vertical movement when running at seven to 12 miles per hour than marathoners. However, such speeds are well below those required during middle-distance races and probably do not represent the running efficiency of competitors in shorter events of 1,500 meters or less. It is interesting to note that the oxygen consumption at a given running speed is also less for world class middle-distance runners than it is for less successful middle-distance runners.

LIMITS OF OXYGEN DELIVERY

Although it is important for runners to be efficient, the upper limits of energy expenditure are determined by one's capacity for oxygen consumption. Earlier we indicated that successful distance runners are characterized by the ability to consume large amounts of oxygen during exhaustive running ($\dot{V}O_2$max). Higher $\dot{V}O_2$max levels enable runners to use lower percentages of those levels to meet the aerobic energy demands of distance competition and avoid heavily taxing their oxygen transportation systems.

If, for example, two runners having $\dot{V}O_2$max values of 60 ml/kg × min (Runner A) and 70 ml/kg × min (Runner B) were asked to run at a six minute per mile pace, both runners would consume about 50 ml of O_2/kg body wt./min. Because of the difference in their aerobic capacities (60 vs. 70 ml/kg × min), the demands placed on their cardiovascular and muscular systems would be markedly different. Runner A, for example, would be working at 83% of his $\dot{V}O_2$max, whereas runner B would only use 71% of his aerobic capacity. Runner B could sustain that pace for a longer period and feel less distress than runner A.

The fractional use of the aerobic capacity (%$\dot{V}O_2$max) for runners competing at distances of five to 84 kilometers (3.1 to 52.2 miles) has been estimated from treadmill testing. Figure 2-2 illustrates that as the distance of the race increases, runners must work at lower percentages of their $\dot{V}O_2$max. Although there are differences in the shape of this curve, marathoners generally run at speeds that require them to use 75 to 80% $\dot{V}O_2$max during competition. As mentioned earlier, however, elite runners Grete Waitz, Frank Shorter, and Derek Clayton were estimated to use between 85 and 90% $\dot{V}O_2$max during the

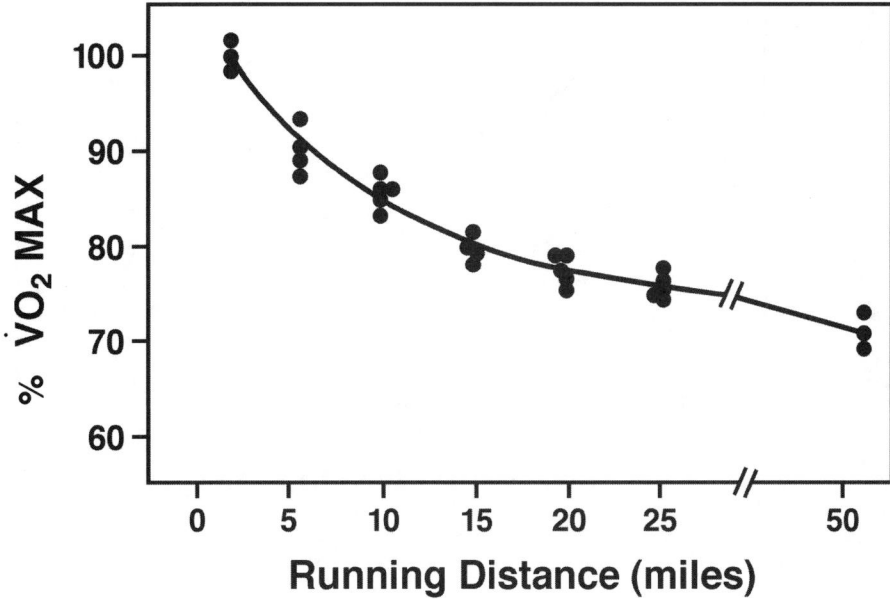

Figure **2-2.** *The average percentage of maximal oxygen uptake (percent* $\dot{V}O_2max$*) used during races from 1,500 meters to 84,000 meters (0.93 to 52.2 miles).*

marathon. Most runners can tolerate this level of effort for distances of only 10 miles or less.

The ability to judge just the right pace depends on a number of sensory inputs, such as muscle tension, respiratory rate, carbon dioxide production and the visual sensation of speed. Through experience, the runner learns to match these sensations with just the right level of energy expenditure.

We studied 16 distance runners in Salford, England where we observed that their percent $\dot{V}O_2max$ during a 10-mile (16.1 kilometer) race ranged from 82 to 92% with an average of 86%. Though the runners' times in the 10-mile run were not related to either the percent $\dot{V}O_2max$ during the run or the amount of lactate in the blood after the run. The best predictor of their performance was $\dot{V}O_2max$. As you can see in Figure 2-3, those with the highest max $\dot{V}O_2$ ran the 10 miles in less than 50 minutes, whereas those with maximal values of 50–55 ml/kg × min were nearly 20 minutes slower for the run.

It has been suggested that the level of blood lactic acid (lactate) during submaximal exercise may be a good indicator of endurance capacity. Terms such as "anaerobic threshold," "aerobic threshold," and the "onset of blood lactate accumulation (OBLA)," are used to describe the sudden change in respiration and lactate accumulation during progressive increments in running speed. Since lactate tends to be produced by the muscles when they are unable to acquire sufficient oxygen to produce energy aerobically, its accumulation in the blood is considered to be an indicator of the pace that the runner can tolerate during long runs.

Figure 2-4 illustrates the relationship between blood lactate levels and running speeds for an elite marathoner and a good collegiate cross-country runner.

r = - 0·91
Test Race = *
V̇O₂ MAX (ml/kg x min)
80
70
60
50
45
50
55
60
65
Time for 10 Mile Run (min)

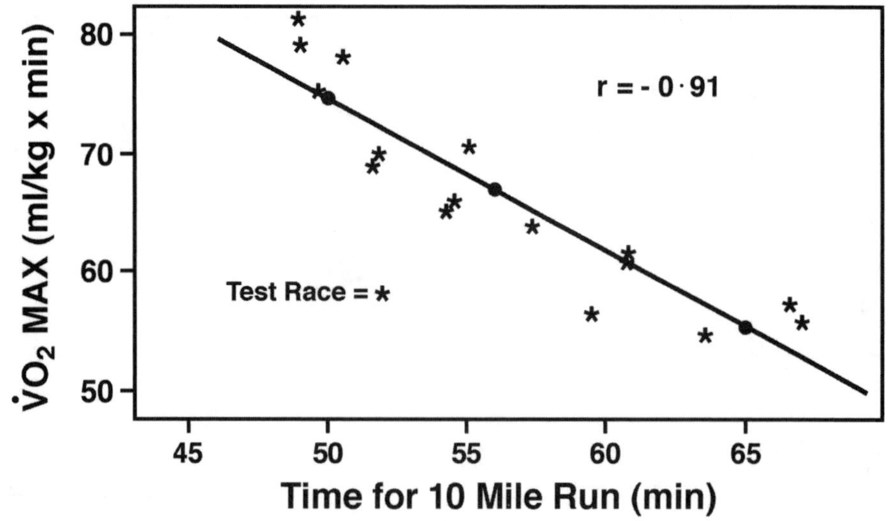

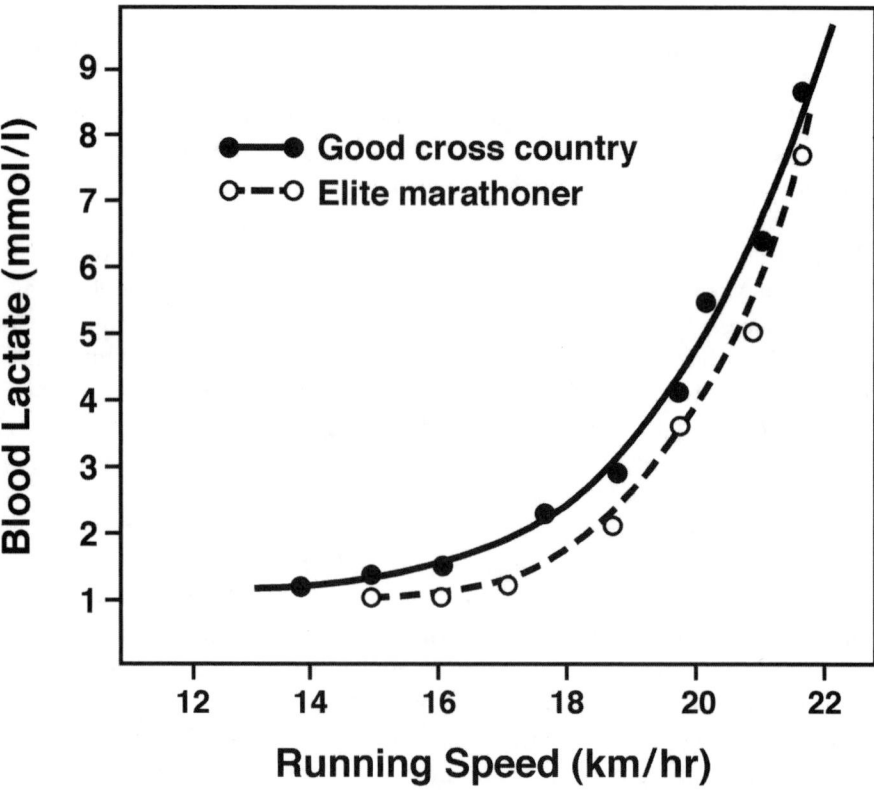

Figure 2-3. *Relationship between time during a 10-mile race and the runners' $\dot{V}O_2max$ (ml/kg × min).*

Good cross country
Elite marathoner
Blood Lactate (mmol/l)
9
8
7
6
5
4
3
2
1
12
14
16
18
20
22
Running Speed (km/hr)

Figure 2-4. *The relationship between running speed and the onset of blood lactic acid accumulation (OBLA). Note that lactate changes very little at the slower speeds, but begins to rise rapidly when the runner's pace exceeds 16 kilometers per hour (6 min per mile).*

Whereas the cross-country runner is able to run comfortably at speeds below six minutes per mile with little accumulation in lactate, the marathoner can run at nearly five minutes per mile before there is any appreciable lactate accumulation. Such laboratory measurements have been used to predict performance and to select an optimal training pace. Additional attention will be given to this topic in the discussion on training in Chapter 4.

Runners seldom maintain a steady pace throughout a race, especially when the terrain is hilly. Estimates of average energy expenditures during competition are a bit misleading, because it is logistically difficult to obtain measurements from runners during competition. One exception was a Swedish study in 1972, which measured oxygen consumption in runners during a 30-kilometer cross-country race. The results revealed that the percent $\dot{V}O_2$max varied from 76% during downhill running to 90% during uphill running. During those same periods heart rates averaged 174 and 180 beats/min, respectively, compared to the subjects' maximal heart rate of 189 beats/min.

Despite the runner's option to reduce the pace to compensate for variations in terrain, a hilly course may be more costly than a level one. This fact was confirmed by a study in 1970, which demonstrated that when men ran on a 6% incline (six meters of vertical climb per 100 meters of horizontal distance) at an eight minute per mile pace, they consumed 35% more energy than they did during level running. Running down a similar grade, however, only reduced the energy demands by 24%. Despite a potential balance between uphill and downhill running, a hilly course will cost significantly more than a level race course.

Some runners, however, are considerably more efficient in running up and down various inclines than their competitors. In the same study, the individual oxygen requirements varied from 50 to 61 ml/kg × min on the incline, and from 27 to 34 ml/kg × min on the down slope. Simply because a runner is efficient while running on the level, does not mean that he or she will be efficient while running uphill or downhill.

Variations in terrain can also affect the stress placed on the different leg muscles. When a runner was made to run uphill or downhill on a treadmill at 70% $\dot{V}O_2$max for two hours, we noted that the thigh muscle (vastus lateralis) was notably more active than it was during level running. This suggests that it is important to include hill running in training programs to prepare for the specific demands of road and cross-country competition.

A small amount of energy is needed to move the body through the air, a major factor when there is a headwind. Early studies suggested that during distance running, roughly 5 to 8% of the energy spent is needed to overcome the resistance to movement through still air. The energy cost of running at a constant speed against the wind was found to increase as the head wind increased. When someone runs on a track in calm air, the difference in oxygen uptake will increase with the cube of the running velocity. The difference in oxygen consumption can, therefore, be computed by the equation:

$$\dot{V}o_{2\text{-diff}} = 0.002 \times \dot{V}^3$$

Where $\dot{V}o_{2\text{-diff}}$ is the increase in oxygen uptake in liters per minute and V is the velocity of the air in meters per second.

As an example, running into a 10 mile per hour (4.44 meters per second) headwind would mean an increase in oxygen uptake ($\dot{V}o_{2\text{-diff}}$) of 0.18 liters per minute ($0.002 \times 4.44^3 = 0.18$). If the runner were traveling at eight minutes per mile where the oxygen requirements were about 2.50 liters per minute in still air, the added headwind would increase the cost of running to 2.68 liters per minute, a 7% increase in energy demand.

At the highest running speeds, variations in body contour and clothing have a dramatic effect on air resistance and energy expenditure. These findings demonstrate that a considerable advantage may be gained by runners who select to run in the "aerodynamic shadow" (drafting) of their competition.

FUELS FOR THE FIRE

The production of energy by the leg muscles depends on the availability of the foods we eat and fuels stored in the body as carbohydrates and fats. As illustrated in Figure 2-5, these fuels are broken down in the presence of oxygen by the mitochondria, the powerhouses of the cell, to produce the ATP for muscular work. These fuels are stored in the muscles and liver as glycogen (carbohydrate) and in the fat cells as triglyceride. The storage of body fat is very large, but the supply of carbohydrates is limited.

The electron micrograph (Figure 2-6) offers a view inside a single muscle fiber, exposing the contractile filaments that make the muscle shorten (C), the mitochondria (A), and glycogen granules (B). During exercise the number of glycogen granules is gradually reduced, as a result of their breakdown to produce energy.

As early as the 1920s experts knew that carbohydrates were the preferred fuel for muscles during distance running. Although the muscles generally use a mixture of carbohydrates and fats to produce the energy for muscular effort, greater demands are placed on blood glucose and muscle glycogen than on the body's stored fat.

At the onset of exercise, muscle glycogen is the primary source of carbohydrate used for energy. We illustrated this point by having a runner perform a three hour treadmill run at a pace that equaled his best marathon time. Biopsies taken from his calf muscles at intervals during the run showed a rapid decline in glycogen. Although the test was run at a steady pace, the rate of muscle glycogen use was greatest during the first 90 minutes of running. Thereafter, the use of glycogen slowed as it approached zero. The runner felt only moderately stressed

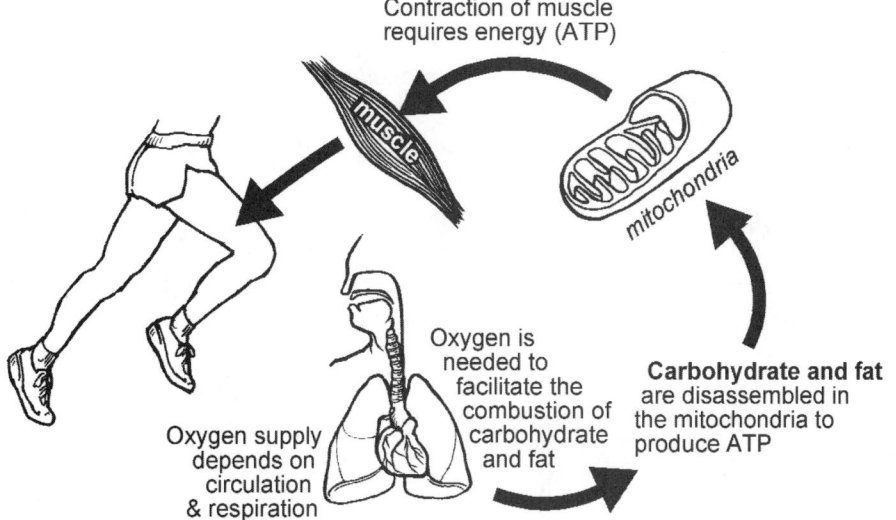

Contraction of muscle
requires energy (ATP)

muscle

mitochondria

Oxygen is
needed to
facilitate the
combustion of
carbohydrate
and fat

Carbohydrate and fat
are disassembled in
the mitochondria to
produce ATP

Oxygen supply
depends on
circulation
& respiration

*Figure 2-5. The
interaction of
respiration, circulation,
and the energy-
producing mechanisms
needed by the muscle
during distance
running. The oxygen
transported to the
muscle is used by the
mitochondria of the
muscle to breakdown
fat and carbohydrate,
producing ATP for
contraction.*

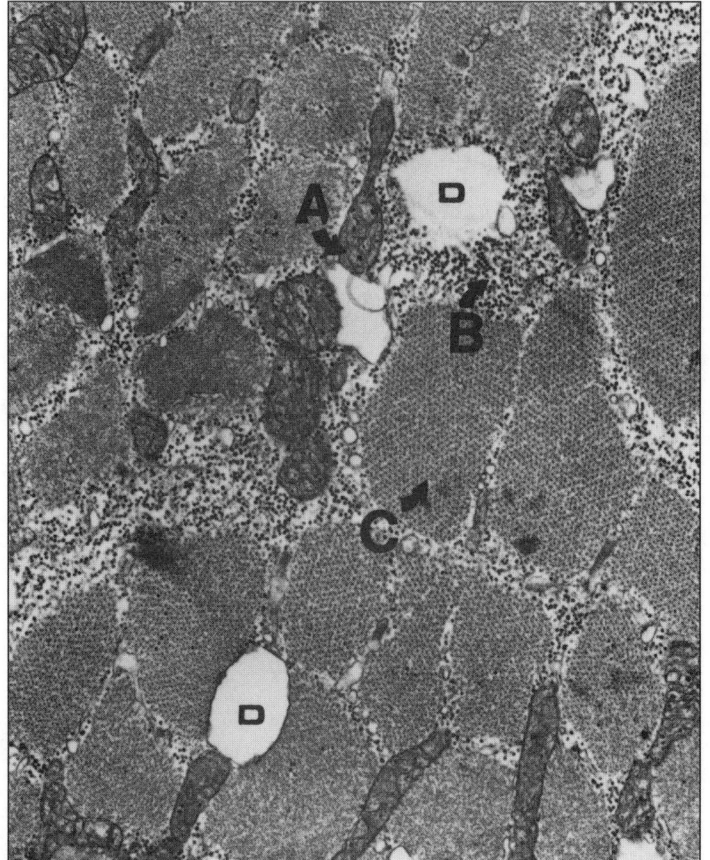

*Figure 2-6.
Electronmicrograph
(20,000 × magnification)
looking inside a single
muscle fiber. If the
contractile filaments,
actin and myosin (C),
are to perform the work
of contraction, then they
must be provided with
ATP which is produced
within the mitochondria
(A). The carbohydrate
stored in the muscle
fiber are glycogen
granules (B). Fat is also
stored as droplets within
the fiber (D).*

during the early part of the run, when his rate of muscle glycogen use was most rapid. Not until muscle glycogen was nearly depleted did he experience severe fatigue (note: and demand considerable financial reward before agreeing to finish the trial).

Runners have no way of knowing what type of fuels their muscles are using or how rapidly the muscles are depleting glycogen. Since the rate of muscle glycogen use increases somewhat in proportion to running speed, a fast pace in the early part of a race may lead to glycogen depletion and premature exhaustion. A runner must carefully choose the correct pace for the length of the run. When muscle glycogen levels are very low, running speed is reduced and exhaustion is not far away.

In the late 1930s Scandinavian physiologists showed that at exercise levels below 95% of a runner's $\dot{V}O_2max$, both carbohydrates and fats are used as fuels. Above this intensity, however, carbohydrates are used almost exclusively.

Although studies with cyclists showed that muscle glycogen was depleted from the thigh muscles after one hour of exercise at 80% $\dot{V}O_2max$, runners have shown that total depletion of muscle glycogen seldom occurs at the end of races which demanded the same intensity of effort. After a 10-mile run of roughly 60 minutes, for example, glycogen was still available in the thigh muscles (vastus lateralis). We could interpret this to mean that exhaustion in running is not related to the depletion of muscle glycogen. But, there are two other possible explanations for the discrepancy between muscular exhaustion in cycling and running.

First, the thigh muscles may be more heavily used during cycling than running. Exhaustion in distance running may deplete other leg muscles more than is reflected by the samples taken from the thigh. To test this theory, we had men run on the level, uphill, and downhill for two hours and obtained biopsies from the thigh (vastus lateralis), deep calf (soleus) and superficial calf (gastrocnemius) muscles at rest and after 70 and 120 minutes of running (Figure 2-7). Greater amounts of glycogen were used from the gastrocnemius and soleus than the vastus lateralis. This suggests that the thigh muscles are not a representative muscle group for study during exhaustive running. Only during uphill and downhill running is the vastus lateralis required to use glycogen at rates approximating those used by the muscles of the lower leg. Even under these circumstances, the glycogen content in the vastus lateralis did not approach zero, despite extreme exhaustion.

A second possibility might explain the lack of complete muscle glycogen depletion at exhaustion during distance running. In 1972, we studied the use of glycogen in slow-twitch (ST) and fast-twitch (FTa and FTb) muscle fibers in runners before and after a 30-kilometer cross-country race. Microscopic examination of these muscle samples (Figure 2-8) revealed that the glycogen content of the slow-twitch fibers was nearly exhausted, while the fast-twitch fibers still contained considerable quantities. This demonstrates that the slow-twitch fibers are the muscle cells most heavily used during this type of running. When the

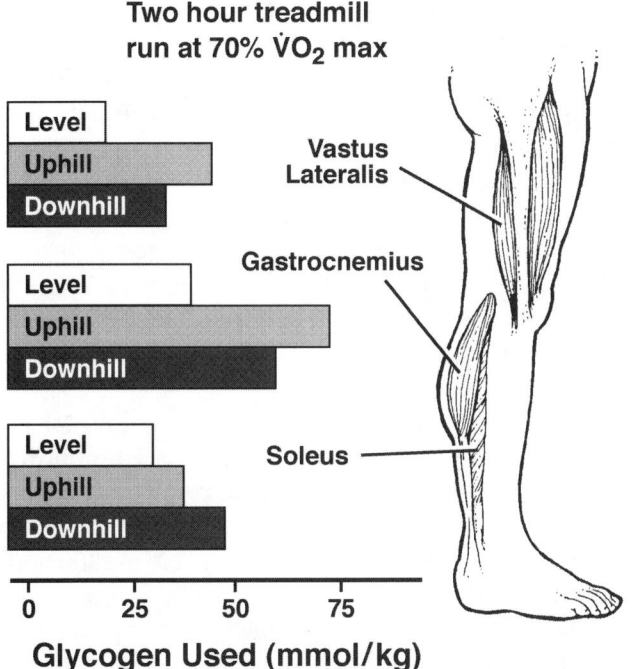

Figure 2-7. *Amount of glycogen used from the thigh (vastus lateralis) and calf (soleus and gastrocnemius) muscles during level, uphill, and downhill running for two hours at 70% of $\dot{V}O_2max$.*

Two hour treadmill run at 70% $\dot{V}O_2$ max

Level
Uphill
Downhill

Level
Uphill
Downhill

Level
Uphill
Downhill

Vastus Lateralis
Gastrocnemius
Soleus

0   25   50   75

Glycogen Used (mmol/kg)

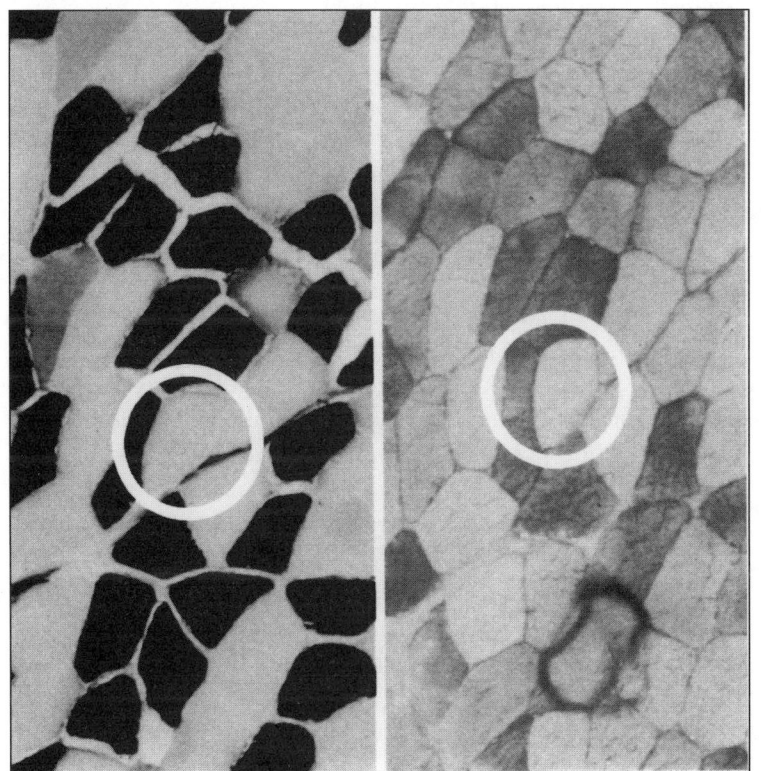

Figure 2-8. *In the left panel is a fiber type stain showing slow-twitch (circled) and fast-twitch muscle fibers. In the right panel is a corresponding muscle glycogen stain. The circled fiber is the same slow-twitch fiber shown in the left panel. As can be seen, the slow-twitch fibers contain little to no muscle glycogen.*

slow-twitch fibers have relinquished their glycogen stores, the fast-twitch fibers are apparently unable to generate enough tension and/or cannot be easily recruited to compensate for the exhausted slow-twitch fibers. As a result, the runner finds each stride progressively more difficult. This selective depletion of muscle glycogen is undoubtedly the cause of the muscle distress often described by runners during the final stage of races like the marathon.

Muscle glycogen alone cannot provide all of the carbohydrate needed for a long-distance run. The liver breaks down glycogen to provide a constant supply of glucose in the blood. In the early stages of exercise, energy production uses relatively small amounts of blood glucose, but in the later stages, blood glucose may make a large contribution. The longer the exercise period, the greater the glucose output from the liver.

Exercising muscles also show a greater uptake and use of glucose with increasing periods of exercise. Since the liver has a limited supply of glycogen and is unable to produce glucose rapidly, blood glucose levels may begin to decrease when the muscle uptake becomes greater than the liver's output. We have sampled blood from runners at each five-mile point in a marathon and observed that glucose gradually declined until the level was clinically abnormal near the finish of the race. Similar findings were reported as early as 1924, which led to the generalization that low blood glucose may be one of the factors responsible for exhaustion during distance running.

Recent studies do not show consistent support for this concept. Measurements of blood glucose during 1.5 to 4 hours of treadmill running have shown a number of cases of extremely low blood glucose without symptoms of fatigue or exhaustion. This does not mean that low blood glucose is not a cause for fatigue. On the contrary, when the glucose supply from the blood is low, muscles must rely more on their own carbohydrate reserves. As a result, muscle glycogen is depleted more rapidly, which leads to inevitable exhaustion.

Both lipids (fat) and amino acids (protein) have been shown to serve as significant energy sources during long runs. Although protein is the major building block of body tissues, it also contributes to the muscle's energy needs as a source of fuel for glucose production in the liver. Estimates of protein use during exercise suggest that as much as 9% of the total energy expended during a marathon race may be derived from amino acids. Some of the amino acids like alanine may be used by the liver to form glucose, which is subsequently used by the muscles. Though the muscles may use protein in this indirect way to get energy, they do not have the capacity to use amino acids directly.

Runners draw on fat deposits inside and outside the muscle fibers during races longer than 10 kilometers (6.2 miles). Up to that distance, runners rely primarily on carbohydrates exclusively, since they are working at more than 90 to 95% $\dot{V}O_2$max values. By measuring the exchange of carbon dioxide and oxygen in a runner's respired air, we can estimate the percentage of energy derived from both fat and carbohydrates.

During a two-hour treadmill test at 65% $\dot{V}O_2$max, we have observed a decrease in the ratio between carbon dioxide and oxygen (RER = $VCo_2/\dot{V}O_2$max) from 0.88 at 10 minutes of exercise to 0.80 at 120 minutes. A conversion table tells us that with these RER values fats were contributing about 39% of the total energy for running at 10 minutes and 67% during the final minutes of exercise. This increase in fat use seems to be related to a rise in blood free fatty acids (FFA), a simple form of fat released from the breakdown of triglyceride in the fat cells.

This shift toward a greater reliance on fat as an energy source was profoundly demonstrated in our studies with an ultra-distance runner, Tom Osler, who ran-walked-rested for 70 hours. Although he consumed food ad labium throughout the trial, there was a gradual shift toward greater and greater use of fat. Over the final hours of the exercise, fat was contributing 90 to 100% of all the energy he needed.

Although it is well known that fats are stored in the skeletal muscles as triglyceride, the importance of fat during distance running is not fully understood. Studies in the early 1970s demonstrated that muscle triglyceride is a major energy source during exercise. The unique ability of slow-twitch muscle fibers to use oxygen allows them to derive a larger part of their energy from fat than the fast-twitch fibers. Since slow-twitch fibers are the ones most frequently used during endurance training and competition, it is not surprising to find that they also have larger storages of triglyceride. In Chapter 4 we will discuss how endurance training tends to increase the storage of both triglyceride and glycogen.

CARDIOVASCULAR RESPONSES

Since distance running is primarily an aerobic form of exercise, great demands are placed on the cardiovascular system, which transports oxygen and fuels to the working muscles and removes wastes produced during energy production. As a measure of the stress imposed on the heart and vascular system, experts have estimated that marathoners performing a 2 h: 26 min marathon would maintain an average cardiac output of 26.5 l/min. Since these same runners had a maximal cardiac output of 28.8 l/min, it seems that these highly trained runners can exercise for nearly two and one-half hours while stressing their cardiovascular systems at 92% of its full capacities. The amount of blood being pumped with each beat (stroke volume) would average about 149 ml/beat (5 oz) at a heart rate of 178 beats/min, which would be near the runner's maximum of 153 ml/beat and 188 beats/min, respectively.

These average values obtained during prolonged exercise may be somewhat misleading, since cardiac output, stroke volume, and heart rate are not constant throughout a race. Swedish physiologists have shown that during more than three hours of exercise at 75% Vo_2max (approximate marathon pace), cardiac output rose 10% with a 5% increase in oxygen uptake. The major circulatory changes during this exercise were a 15% progressive rise in heart rate and a 12% fall in stroke volume. The causes for these changes are not known, though some have speculated that the rise in heart rate and fall in stroke volume may be caused by a rise in body temperature with an increase in blood flow to the skin. When body temperature is elevated, as is the case in distance running, central blood volume and stroke volume fall, thereby forcing the heart rate to rise in an effort to keep the runner's cardiac output constant.

To complicate the issue even more, during the initial minutes of running, the water in blood plasma decreases. This change in plasma volume is due to a rise in the pressure of the small blood vessels within the muscle, which results in a shift in fluids from the blood into and around the muscle fibers. The effect of this plasma water loss is a relative increase in hematocrit (percent of blood composed of red blood cells) and hemoglobin concentration.

The major change in the cardiovascular system during long-distance races appears to be a gradual relaxing of the blood vessels in the skin and other tissues, causing blood to shift from the central vessels to the periphery. Since the normal operations of the heart are reduced throughout a long run, cardiac output is maintained by an increased heart rate. It is difficult to determine whether the heart muscle actually fatigues during long duration running, but in a healthy heart it is unlikely. Nevertheless, with exhaustion, stimulation of the smooth muscles surrounding the arterial vessels may constrict the vessels and reduce blood flow to less active regions of the body such as the digestive organs. This may explain the pallor and gastrointestinal distress sometimes seen at exhaustion.

From a practical point of view, the simplest method for monitoring the stress of exercise is to measure your heart rate during or immediately after running. Since modern technology has created several commercial monitors, runners can observe their heart rates during training runs and competition. But you should know that heart rate responses to exercise are an individual thing. Only experience with a heart rate monitor during training runs of different intensities and durations will provide you with your profile.

Although several formulas have been suggested to indicate the "ideal" heart rate to achieve optimal conditioning, the preferred heart rate during training is usually in the range of 130 to 150 beats per minute for men, and 150 to 170 beats per minute for women. Of course these values will vary widely, depending on the running pace, physical condition, and individual differences in maximal heart rate. Individuals with unusually low or high maximal heart rates may be proportionately lower or higher during training runs. Although there are prediction tables to estimate your maximal heart rate based on age, these tables can be grossly in error for some individuals. If you have a method of monitoring your heart rate during exercise, maximal heart rate can be determined by performing a four- to-five-minute maximal run. The heart rate recorded during the last 30 to 60 seconds of the run or within 15 seconds after the end of the run will reflect the maximal rate. Such information will help to judge the optimal stimulus for training and to prevent overtraining

RESPIRATION: A BREATHTAKING EVENT

To accommodate the high rate of oxygen consumption demanded during distance running, large volumes of air must be delivered to the lungs. Breathing is probably the most obvious subjective indicator you use to gauge your pace and level of distress. Although the volume of air breathed per minute is not directly proportional to the amount of oxygen being consumed by the body, most runners adjust the running pace to permit a tolerable level of respiratory distress.

The air we breathe is a mixture of gases, about 21% of which is oxygen. After we inhale the gases into the lungs, some of the oxygen is taken up by the blood to replace that being used by the muscle and other tissues. At the same time, carbon dioxide (CO_2), the by-product of aerobic energy production, is released into the lungs' gases to be exhaled. Consequently, the air leaving the lungs has less oxygen (15 to 17%) and more carbon dioxide (3 to 5%).

While the average person may breathe approximately five to six liters of air per minute at rest, the volume may exceed 150 liters per minute during intense running. In the late 1960s we studied a group of runners during a simulated 10,000-meter run. These runners were able to breathe between 120 and 145 liters of air per minute for more than 20 minutes of the run. Such values are unusually large, since these men were relatively small, averaging 143 pounds in weight. Other non-endurance trained athletes are only able to breathe such large volumes for one or two minutes of voluntary effort or during the final seconds of an exhaustive exercise bout. One of the unique adaptations to training among distance runners is the ability of the respiratory muscles to sustain a high breathing rate and volume for prolonged periods.

One might ask the question, "Does breathing become a limiting factor during long-distance running?" At least two points should be considered in answering.

First, the work of breathing places heavy demands on the muscles that expand and contract the chest wall. Though the oxygen consumed by the respiratory muscles under resting conditions is small (about 1% of the body's total energy need), the cost of breathing becomes progressively greater with increasing levels of effort. Since the actual efficiency of the respiratory muscles cannot be measured, it is impossible to be precise in estimates of the energy needed to ventilate the lungs. During distance races, where the respiratory volume may average 100 to 120 liters per minute, as much as 9% of the energy used by the body will be needed for respiration. In any event, though the work of breathing increases with increased effort, respiratory ventilation is probably not a limiting factor in long-distance races except perhaps at high altitude.

The second consideration is the problem of maintaining normal oxygen and carbon dioxide concentrations in the blood. Previous studies have demonstrated that arterial oxygen content remains relatively constant at various levels of exercise. However, in athletes with breathing volumes of 120 to 150 liters per minute, a fall in arterial oxygen content has been observed at exhaustion. Since long-distance runners or marathoners seldom tax their respiratory systems to the maximum during competition, it is unlikely that the diffusion of gases between the lung and blood will become limiting. This may not be the case, however, in shorter races of 5,000 to 10,000 meters. Little scientific evidence is available to determine the effects of such high-intensity running on the arterial oxygen content during the final stages of such competition, when many runners experience extreme respiratory distress.

Subjective reports of breathing distress near the end of marathon and longer races are not uncommon. Considering the constant, intense demands placed on the respiratory muscles throughout such events, these muscles may simply be experiencing the order of fatigue confronting the leg muscles, glycogen depletion. The task of ventilating the lungs may become more difficult, leading to a sensation of respiratory resistance. After many hours of intense respiratory effort, there also may be some swelling of the bronchioles in the respiratory pathway, which would cause some resistance to breathing and lead to additional respiratory muscle fatigue. Further studies are needed on the importance of breathing to distance running performance.

Most runners monitor various senses of effort, especially breathing, in order to judge their pace. Aside from the visual clues of the speed of movement and the sensations of muscular effort, the runner has little to directly indicate the rate of energy expenditure.

Breathing rate and depth are the best physiological guides to monitor pace. Even during running in hot weather or at high altitude, the signs of labored breathing reflect the level of stress imposed on the cardiovascular and energy system and serve as a warning of overstress.

BY-PRODUCTS OF RUNNING

In the process of using fuels to produce energy aerobically, the muscles generate a number of waste products, including carbon dioxide, heat, and lactic acid (lactate). Since excessive amounts of these by-products can impair normal muscle function, they must be removed from the cell as quickly as possible. Fortunately, most of these by-products of energy production diffuse rapidly out of the cells and into the blood. When an individual runs at an easy submaximal pace, the circulatory system is able to transport carbon dioxide and heat to the lungs and skin where they can be dissipated, minimizing build-ups in the blood.

By-products such as lactic acid, however, are not so easily eliminated and accumulate rapidly during intense effort. Since lactic acid is formed only when the muscles produce energy anaerobically, one would not expect it to accumulate to any degree in distance running. Although this is the case in most relatively easy training runs and long races, a sizeable amount of lactate may appear in the blood and muscles during shorter events of 10 miles or less.

During the initial seconds or minutes of a race, a runner's circulatory and respiratory systems cannot adjust to the sudden burst of energy demanded by the muscles. The immediate oxygen requirements may be far greater than the circulatory system can supply, forcing the muscles to derive some energy anaerobically, without sufficient oxygen. Consequently, the runner incurs an oxygen debt with significant lactate accumulation. The muscles and blood become more acid, a condition incompatible with the operation of the cells.

The indication of fluid acidity and alkalinity used to assess body fluids is termed "pH," which is based on a 14 point scale. A solution that is neither acid nor alkaline, such as distilled water, has a pH of roughly 7.0, whereas more acid solutions have lower values, nearing zero.

Arterial blood and resting muscles normally have pH values of 7.4 and 7.1, respectively, slightly on the alkaline side. During hard running, muscle pH may drop to 6.8 or lower, which results in a lowering of blood pH to approximately 7.1. In exhaustive sprint events of 400 meters, muscle lactate may rise from a resting level of 1.0 mmoles of lactate/kg of muscle to 25, with a subsequent decrease in muscle pH to 6.5. Subsequent diffusion of this lactate into the blood causes the blood pH to drop from 7.4 to 6.8 or lower.

Since body tissues can only operate optimally within a very narrow range of pH, such large changes in muscle and blood lactate and pH have a dramatic effect on performance. Increased acidity impairs the operation of the mitochondria, limiting the muscle's ability to produce energy. In addition, the contractile processes of the muscle begin to fail, reducing the tension developed by the muscle. Such changes result in a shortening of the runner's stride and an inability to maintain even a slow speed. It is important to realize, however, that such drastic changes in muscle and blood pH only occur in events that result in large accumulations of lactic acid, which is not the case in long distance running (Figure 2-9).

As an example, blood lactate at the end of various distance races is only slightly above the resting levels after the marathon, but extremely high after races as short as one mile. There are two possible explanations.

First, the longer the race, the smaller the percent $\dot{V}O_2$max used during the run. Consequently, energy can be produced almost exclusively by aerobic means, with little lactate production. Secondly, the lactate produced in the early stages of a long run may be removed by less active tissues, including the liver, kidney, and inactive muscles, even during the exercise. It has been shown that the lactate produced during an hour of exercise reaches a peak concentration in the blood during the first 10 minutes of running. Approximately half of that, however, is removed by the end of 30 minutes of running. This suggests that

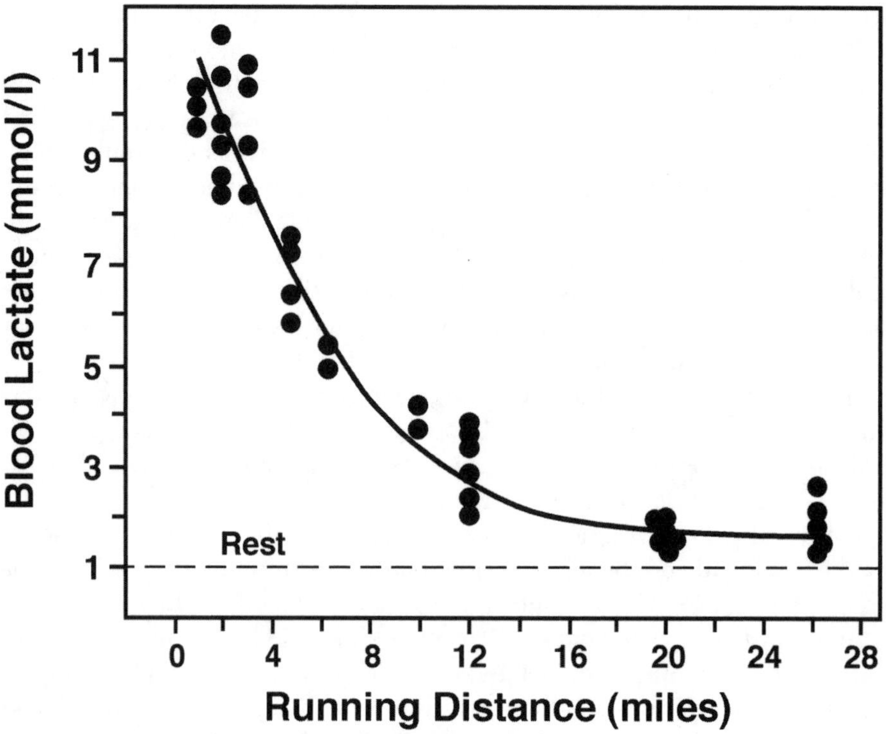

Figure 2-9. *Blood lactate concentrations after races of from one to 26 miles. Note the greatest lactate levels are in the shorter events, whereas the values after marathon races are only slightly above the resting levels.*

changes in blood lactate levels and pH are seldom responsible for the fatigue commonly experienced during races longer than 10 kilometers.

Another common misconception of some runners is that lactic acid causes muscle soreness. In light of the knowledge that little or no lactate is produced during the marathon, an almost purely aerobic event, the leg soreness cannot be attributed to lactate. Theoretically, there is no justification for this belief, since lactate has no properties that could induce pain and tightness. Some new theories concerning muscle soreness and tissue damage will be discussed in Chapter 4 in the section on "Overtraining."

CHANGES IN BLOOD DURING LONG RUNS

Exercising muscles consume greater amounts of glucose during longer running periods. You will recall that the longer the period of exercise, the greater the liver's glucose output. When the muscles' demands for glucose are greater than the liver's output, however, blood glucose levels may fall from the normal level of 5 mmol/l of blood to less than 3. Since blood glucose serves as the primary source of energy for the nervous system, low blood glucose (hypoglycemia) may be one factor responsible for intolerable sensations of fatigue experienced during the final stages of very long races.

As mentioned earlier, free fatty acids provide a large part of the energy during long races like the marathon. Runners do not reap the full benefits of fat energy until they have been running for 30 minutes or longer. This shift toward the use of fat is indicated by a rising level of free fatty acids in plasma, with a concomitant increase in plasma glycerol, a by-product of the breakdown of triglyceride. Fat provides an alternate source of energy and spares the potential exhaustion of muscle glycogen stores during endurance exercise.

There are a number of other changes in the composition of blood during distance running, but none of them seem to impose any risk to the runner's health. Despite relatively large changes in blood proteins during distance running, there is no evidence to suggest that there are any health risks associated with the distress of fatigue. Although special proteins and enzymes play important roles in the energy mechanisms of the muscle, the significance of their increases in blood may simply reflect some injury to the muscle and/or the result of high rates of metabolism in the liver and muscles. As we will discuss in Chapter 4, there is substantial evidence indicating some damage to the muscle membranes during long runs, which seem to explain how these proteins leak into the blood. The significance of this muscle trauma appears to be only temporary and quite reversible.

As previously discussed, there is a rapid movement of water from plasma into the working musculature. This loss of water from the blood causes many of the dissolved particles in the blood to become concentrated, since most of them do not move out of the vessels as rapidly as water. We may see a marked increase in the concentration of such plasma particles as cholesterol and protein, even though the total amount of these items in circulation does not change.

RUNNING HOT

Probably no single factor poses a greater threat to the distance runner's health and performance than overheating. Since much of the energy generated by a muscle is not used for contractions, most of the energy is degraded to the lowest form of energy, heat. Consequently, the internal heat of the muscle rises rapidly during exercise, reaching temperatures of 106 to 108°F. In order to cool the muscle, the internal heat is transferred to the blood passing through the small vessels (capillaries) that surround the muscle fibers. As a result, the muscle heat raises the temperature of the blood and the internal temperature of the body.

While moderate changes in body temperature are tolerated, fevers of 104°F or higher can affect the nervous system and the body's mechanisms of temperature regulation. The removal of heat from the body is regulated by the hypothalamus, a small mass of nervous tissue seated in the base of the brain. Functioning as a thermostat, the hypothalamus triggers a sweating response and helps to direct blood flow to the skin in an effort to dissipate the excess body heat. Although surprisingly effective, this system of cooling is not without limitations, and often it is no match for the high rate of heat produced during running.

One of the primary responsibilities of the circulatory system is to transport heat from the muscles to the surface of the body where the heat can be transferred to the environment. Since the volume of blood is limited, exercise poses a complex problem for the circulatory system. During exercise, a large part of the cardiac output must be shared by the skin and working muscles an increase in the demand for flow to one tissue will automatically decrease flow to the other.

Any factor that tends to overload the cardiovascular system or interfere with the transfer of heat from the body to the environment will drastically impair the distance runner's performance and increase the risk of overheating. Running at a fast pace, for example, will require more oxygen and blood flow to the muscles, with a concomitantly greater rate of muscle heat production. Despite this increase in heat production, blood flow to the skin must decrease, resulting in an inability to move the heat to the shell of the body. Fast running in warm weather also tends to overload the circulatory system, produce greater heat, and reduce the ability to deliver muscle heat to the skin. This causes greater rise in body temperature.

Under resting conditions the amount of heat produced by the body is relatively small (about 1.5 kilocalories per minute) compared to that generated during distance running (15-20 kilocalories per minute). Whereas excess heat loss at rest is accomplished via radiation or infrared rays, conduction, and convection; roughly 80% of the heat loss during exercise is accomplished through sweat evaporation. With as little as one hundredth of a degree increase in blood temperature, the hypothalamus stimulates the sweat glands in the skin to release sweat, moistening the skin surface. Using the heat delivered to the skin by the blood, sweat is converted from a liquid into a gas. Unless this conversion takes place, little or no heat can be dissipated, and the body begins to store heat at a dangerous rate. When the air is humid, for example, it is nearly saturated with water and cannot absorb the water of sweat. As a result, little body heat can be lost and the runner may develop a dangerously high fever.

A number of studies have reported rectal temperatures higher than 104°F after marathon races conducted on moderately warm days. Following a 10,000-meter race in the heat (85°F, 80% relative humidity, and bright sun) we recorded a rectal temperature of 109.5°F in a 40-year-old man who collapsed only 100 yards from the finish. Without proper medical attention, such fevers result in permanent brain damage and in some cases death. Fortunately, this man was rapidly cooled with ice and recovered without complications. Body temperature during distance running is directly dependent on running speed, gross body weight, or both. Heavier individuals would run a higher risk of overheating than lighter athletes when they are running at the same pace.

There is little we can do about the environmental conditions, but it is obvious that runners must slow down to reduce heat production and the risk of overheating. All runners and race promoters should be able to recognize the symptoms of a high internal fever. There is a fair relationship between subjective sensations and the runner's body temperature. The following are some of the symptoms associated with overheating. Although we are seldom concerned with rectal temperatures of 101 to 104°F at the end of prolonged exercise, a runner who has a throbbing pressure in his head and chills should realize that he is rapidly approaching a dangerous stage that could prove fatal if he continues to run.

Heat stroke, the result of a high internal temperature, is the major threat to the well-trained, highly motivated distance runner. Some guidelines to follow for the prevention of such heat-related injuries are as follows:

1. Distance races of greater than 10 kilometers should not be conducted when the combination of air temperature, humidity, and sun raise the WBGT temperature above 82°F. This combination of environmental heat stress conditions (WBGT) can be calculated as follows:

   $$WBGT = 0.7(TWB) + 0.2(TG) = 0.1(TDB)$$

   where TWB = temperature of wet bulb; TG = temperature of black globe; and TDB = temperature of dry bulb

2. Summer events should be scheduled before 8 a.m. or after 6 p.m. to minimize the radiant heat from the sun.
3. An adequate supply of water or other fluids should be available before the race and at two- to three-kilometer intervals during the race. Runners should drink 100 to 200 milliliters at each feeding station.
4. Runners should train adequately for fitness and become heat-acclimatized.
5. Runners should be aware of the early symptoms of heat injury, including dizziness, chilling, headache, and awkwardness.
6. Race sponsors should make prior arrangements with medical personnel to care for heat injuries. Responsible and informed personnel should supervise each feeding station. Organizational personnel should reserve the right to stop runners who exhibit clear signs of heat stroke or heat exhaustion.

Heat exhaustion, although not usually life-threatening, is characterized by dizziness, nausea, weakness, and pale skin that is cool and moist. Unconsciousness often accompanies these symptoms, induced by a sudden pooling of blood in the skin and a drop in blood flow to the brain.

The frequency of **muscle cramping** increases during distance running in the heat. Although such cramping may be the consequence of large water and mineral losses in sweat, the precise cause is not fully understood. As a matter of fact, no conclusive explanations or objective data are available to explain the cause of muscle cramping. Since cramps occur under a wide variety of conditions, during sleep and in exercise, there are probably a number of possible causes.

OPTIMIZING THE USE OF ENERGY FOR RUNNING

The preceding discussion has pointed out some of the costly aspects of distance running and factors that may limit one's performance. Though body weight is one of the most important factors determining the amount of energy needed to run at a given speed, there are marked individual differences in running efficiency. It costs some runners more to run at a given speed than it does others with better technique.

This leads us to wonder why so little effort is made to improve the runner's mechanics. In nearly every other sport, at least part of each training session is directed toward the improvement of skill. This is not the case in distance running. Few runners ever attempt to analyze or improve their running techniques. When we consider the fact that even a 1% decrease in the energy cost of running would improve a three-hour marathoner's time by nearly two minutes, it is surprising that more attention is not given to this aspect of training. Although the biomechanical aspects of running are outside the scope of this book, it is obvious that skill and energy expenditure are important determinants of success in long-distance events.

CLASSIC AND SUGGESTED READINGS

Bergstrom, J. and E. Hultman. A study of the glycogen metabolism during exercise in man. *Scand. J. Clin. Lab. Invest.,* 19:218–228, 1967.

Bergstrom, J., L. Hermansen, E. Hultman and B. Saltin. Diet, muscle glycogen and physical performance. *Acta Physiol. Scand.,* 71:140–150, 1967.

Costill, D. L. Salazar and Clayton: A physiological comparison of the marathon record holders. *The Runner,* 20, March, 1982.

Costill, D. L. Metabolic responses during distance running. *J. Appl. Physiol.,* 28:251–255, 1970.

Costill, D. L. Muscular exhaustion during distance running. *Physician and Sportsmedicine,* 36–41, October 1974.

Costill, D. L., A. Barnett, R. Sharp, W. Fink and A. Katz. Leg muscle pH following sprint running. *Med. Sci. Sports Exer.,* 15:325–329, 1983.

Costill, D. L., E. Jansson, P. D. Gollnick and B. Saltin. Glycogen utilization in leg muscles of men during level and uphill running. *Acta Physiol. Scand.,* 91:475–481, 1974.

Costill, D. L. and E. L. Fox. Energetics of marathon running. *Med. Sci. Sports,* 1:81–86, 1969.

Costill, D. L. and E. Winrow. A comparison of two middle aged ultra-marathon runners. *Res. Quart.*, 41:135–139, 1970.

Costill, D. L., G. Branam, D. Eddy and K. Sparks. Determinants of marathon running success. *Int. Zeitschift fur angewandte Physiol.*, 29:249–254, 1971.

Costill, D. L., H. Thomason and E. Roberts. Fractional utilization of the aerobic capacity during distance running. *Med. Sci. Sports*, 5:248–252, 1973.

Costill, D. L. and J. M. Miller. Nutrition for endurance sport: Carbohydrate and fluid balance. *Int. J. Sports Med.*, 1:2–14, 1980.

Costill, D. L., K. E. Sparks, R. Gregor and C. Turner. Muscle glycogen utilization during exhaustion running. *J. Appl. Physiol.*, 31:353–356, 1971.

Costill, D. L., P. Cleary, W. Fink, C. Foster, J. Ivy and F. Witzmann. Training adaptations in skeletal muscle of juvenile diabetics. *Diabetes*, 28:818–822, 1979.

Costill, D. L., P. D. Gollnick, E. D. Jansson, B. Saltin and E. M. Stein. Glycogen depletion patterns in human muscle fibers during distance running. *Acta Physiol. Scand.*, 89:374–383, 1973.

Costill, D. L., R. Bowers, G. Branam and K. Sparks. Muscle glycogen utilization during prolonged exercise on successive days. *J. Appl. Physiol.*, 31:834–838, 1971.

Costill, D. L., W. F. Kammer and A. Fisher. Fluid ingestion during distance running. *Arch Environ. Health.*, 21:520–525, 1970.

Daniels, J. and N. Oldridge. The effects of alternate exposure to altitude and sea level on world-class middle-distance runners. *Med. Sci. Sports*, 2:107–112, 1970.

Dill, D. B. Oxygen used in horizontal and grade walking and running on the treadmill. *J. Appl. Physiol.*, 20:19–22, 1965.

Farrell, P. A., J. H. Wilmore, E. F. Coyle, J. E. Billing and D. L. Costill. Plasma lactate accumulation and distance running performance. *Med. Sci. Sports*, 11:338–344, 1979.

Fox, E. L. and D. L. Costill. Estimated cardiorespiratory responses during marathon running. *Arch. Environ. Health,* 24:316–324, 1972.

Gisolfi, C. V. and J. Cohen. Relationships among training, heat acclimation and heat tolerance in men and women: the controversy revisited. *Med. Sci. Sports*, 11:56–59,1979.

Gregor, R. A comparison of the energy expenditure during positive and negative grade running. *Master's Thesis, Ball State University, Muncie, Indiana,* 1970.

Hargreaves, M., D. L. Costill, A. Coggan, W. Fink and I. Nishibata. Effect of carbohydrate feedings on muscle glycogen utilization and exercise performance. *Med. Sci.Sports Exer.*, 16:219–222, 1984.

Hermansen, L., E. Hultman and B. Saltin. Muscle glycogen during prolonged severe exercise. *Acta Physiol. Scand.*, 71:129–139, 1967.

Hill, A. V. The air resistance of a runner. *Proc Roy Soc London*, 102:380–385, 1928.

Kew, M. C., I. Bersohn, H. C. Seftel and G. Kent. Liver damage in heat stroke. *Am. J. Med.*, 49:192–202, 1970.

Kielblock, A. J., M. Manjoo and J. Booyen. Creatine phosphokinase and lactate dehydrogenase levels after ultra long-distance running: an analysis of isoenzyme profiles with special reference to indicators of myocardial damages. *S. Afr. Med. J.*, 55:1061–1064, 1979.

Kollias, J., D. L. Moody and E. R. Buskirk. Cross-country running: Treadmill simulation and suggested effectiveness of supplemental treadmill training. *J. Sports Med.*,7:148–154, 1967.

Kollias, J., D. L. Moody and E. R. Buskirk. Cross-country running: Treadmill simulation and suggested effectiveness of supplemental treadmill training. *J. Sports Md. and Phys.*, 7:148–154, 1967.

Levine, S. A., B. Gordon and C. L. Derick. Some changes in the chemical constituents of the blood following a marathon race. *J. Amer. Med. Assoc.*, 82:1778–1779, 1924.

Margaria, R., P. Cerretelli and P. Aghems. Energy cost of running. *J. Appl. Physiol.*, 18:367–370, 1963.

Minard, D. Prevention of heat casualties in Marine Corps Recruits. *Milit. Med.*, 126:261–265, 1961.

Piwonka, R. W., S. Robinson, V. L. Gay and R. S. Manalis. Preacclimatization of men to heat by training. *J. Appl. Physiol.*, 20:379–384, 1965.

Pollock, M. L. Submaximal and maximal working capacity of elite distance runners. *Ann. N.Y Acad. Sci.*, 301:30–44, 1977.

Pugh, L. G. C. Oxygen uptake in track and treadmill running with observations on the effect of air resistance. *J. Physiol.*, 207:825–835, 1970.

Rose, K., J. E. Bousser and K. H. Cooper. Serum enzymes after marathon running. *J. Appl. Physiol.*, 29:355–357, 1970.

Rowell, L. B., H. J. Marx, R. A. Bruce, R. D. Conn and J. Kusumi. Reductions in cardiac output central blood volume with thermal stress in normal men during exercise. *J. Clin. Invest.*, 45:1801–1816, 1966.

Saltin, B. and J. Karlsson. Muscle glycogen utilization during work of different intensities. *Muscle Metabolism During Exercise*, B. Pernow and B. Saltin, ed. New York: Plenum Press, 11:289–300, 1971.

Siegel, A. J., L. M. Silverman and B. L. Holman. Elevated creatine kinase MB isoenzyme levels in marathon runners. *JAMA 246,* :2049–2051, 1981.

Wahren, J., P. Felig, R. Hendler and G. Ahlborg. Glucose and amino acid metabolism during recovery after exercise. *J. Appl. Physiol.*, 34:838–845, 1973.

Wyndham, C. H. and N. B. Strydom. The danger of an inadequate water intake during marathon running. *S. Afr. Med. J.*, 43:893–896, 1969.

Chapter 3
Fueling the Runners Muscles

INTRODUCTION

Aside from the limits imposed by heredity and the adaptations associated with training, no single factor can play a greater role in optimizing performance than diet. Despite the wealth of published information dealing with "proper nutrition," few efforts have been made to describe the nutritional needs and best dietary regimen for the distance runner. Most runners have at one time searched for the "magic foods" that might produce a winning performance. Unfortunately, most dietary regimens for the athlete have been based on anecdotal accounts from other runners, poorly designed nutritional research studies, invalid commercial advertising claims, and the misinterpretation of facts. The following discussion will try to take an objective look at the body's nutrient needs and present the more recent research findings which have direct bearing on running performance.

Historical Note

Likely the most comprehensive study of distance runners occurred in 1975 when Michael Pollock brought 24 of the top U.S. distance runners and sports scientists to the Aerobic Research Institute (Dallas, TX). The New York Academy of Sciences subsequently published the results of that project in 1977.

MUSCLE FUELS

The preceding chapters pointed out that the energy used for all cellular operations is derived from the splitting of a powerful chemical compound known as adenosine triphosphate, or **ATP**. The energy stored in the ATP molecule is created from such fuels as fats, carbohydrates, and proteins. The energy needed to make the muscle fibers shorten cannot be obtained directly from such things as sugar and fat, since they release only small quantities of energy when they are broken down. Nevertheless, by breaking down the chemical structures of those fuels, the small amount of energy can be stockpiled in an ATP molecule, which can release large amounts of energy when its chemical bonds are separated. Consequently, each cell uses the energy stored in ATP as immediate energy for its operation. Without carbohydrates and fats, however, the muscle cannot maintain adequate levels of ATP. Since the mid-1930s we have known that both carbohydrate and fat contribute the primary energy for endurance exercise. Though protein may contribute 6 to 9% of the energy during a long run of 20 miles or more, it is considered to be of only limited importance in ATP production for running performance.

As noted earlier, the fraction of energy derived from carbohydrates during distance running depends on a number of factors including running speed, physical conditioning, environmental temperature, and the pre-exercise diet. Early Scandinavian studies demonstrated that subjects who were fed diets rich in carbohydrates tended to derive a larger amount of their energy from carbohydrate during exercise. Although the underlying cause for this shift toward a higher carbohydrate use following a diet rich in carbohydrates has not been fully explained, such a dietary regimen may inhibit the use of fat. It is important to realize that the muscle has a limited amount of glycogen, and you can't refill the muscle while you are running. So, once you start to run, muscle glycogen is steadily reduced until, at exhaustion, the supply is depleted. Since depletion of muscle and liver glycogen limits performance during distance running, one might question the wisdom of eating a high-carbohydrate diet, which accelerates the combustion of glycogen. This apparent disadvantage is probably offset by the enlarged glycogen reserves that result from the carbohydrate diet, a point to which we will return later.

Blood glucose also serves as a major contributor to the carbohydrate pool. At rest, the uptake of glucose accounts for less than 10% of the total energy used by muscles. During a typical training run, however, the movement of glucose from the blood into the leg muscles may increase 10 to 20 times the resting level. As the duration of exercise is extended, the fraction of energy derived from blood glucose grows and may account for 75 to 90% of the muscles' carbohydrate use. This large drain on blood glucose necessitates an equal increase in liver glucose output to lessen the risk of low blood sugar (hypoglycemia). Since the liver is the major contributor of glucose to blood, the increased demands by muscular activity rapidly reduce liver glycogen stores. During four hours of slow running at 50% of $\dot{V}O_2$max, 75% of a runner's liver glycogen may be removed. As a result, runners who compete in races lasting three or more hours may become hypoglycemic.

As we will discuss later, one of the major adaptations to endurance running is developing a greater capacity to use fat as an energy source. Marathon runners, for example, get more than 75% of their energy from fat oxidation during 60 minutes of running at 70% $\dot{V}O_2$max. Since fat serves as an alternative source of energy for the muscles, anything that might promote its use during distance running tends to spare muscle glycogen and improve endurance.

Thus, optimal distance running performance is strongly influenced by the availability of both carbohydrate and fat. Nutrition plays a central role in both the storage and use of these substances. Though stores of body fat exceed the amounts needed for the longest distance races even the skinniest runner, carbohydrate (glycogen) reserves in the liver and muscles are limited and may not be able to accommodate the requirements of races lasting two to four hours. The distance runner must focus on the intake of carbohydrates to replace tissue glycogen used during training and to promote glycogen storage prior to competition.

RUNNING: THE ATHLETE WITHIN

DIETARY CARBOHYDRATES AND TRAINING

Early studies demonstrated that when men ate a diet containing a normal amount of carbohydrates, about 55% of total calories, their muscles stored approximately 100 mmol of glycogen per kg of muscle. Diets low in carbohydrate, containing less than 15% of total calories, resulted in storage of only 53 mmol/kg of muscle, whereas a rich carbohydrate diet produced a muscle glycogen content of 205 mmol/kg of muscle. When these subjects were asked to exercise to exhaustion at 75% $\dot{V}o_2$max, their exercise times were proportional to the amount of glycogen present in the muscles before the test (Table 3-1). Carbohydrate in the diet clearly has a direct influence on muscle glycogen stores and the runner's ability to train and compete.

Studies from Scandinavia in the mid-1960s indicated that muscle glycogen was restored to muscle within 24 hours after exhaustive exercise if athletes ate a rich carbohydrate diet. Continuing this diet for two additional days elevated the glycogen to twice the pre-exercise level.

More recent studies have shown that glycogen replacement and storage is not so simple. We have observed that seven days after a marathon race in which muscle glycogen dropped from 196 to 26 mmol/kg of muscle, a normal diet and rest restored the glycogen only to 125 (Figure 3-1). We have recorded similarly slow glycogen restoring after exhaustive treadmill running.

This delayed recovery of muscle glycogen seems to be characteristic of distance running, since it does not occur after exhaustive cycling or swimming. Although the cause has not been fully explained, the muscle trauma which occurs in distance running may inhibit the mechanisms normally responsible for the uptake and storage of glucose by the muscle.

Although the amount of carbohydrate in the diet determines, to a large extent, the rate of muscle glycogen storage, there are also some special proteins (enzymes) that combine glucose molecules into glycogen granules. The activity of one such enzyme, glycogen synthase, is very active when muscle glycogen is low, thereby promoting glycogen storage. As the glycogen reserves begin to fill-up, the synthase activity declines, lessening the drive for further glycogen for-

TABLE 3-1. Effects of dietary carbohydrate on muscle glycogen stores and endurance performance.

CHO Intake (GM/24 hr)	Glycogen Content (mmol/kg Muscle)	Exercise Time to Exhaustion (min)
100 gm	53 mmol/kg	57 min
280 gm	100 mmol/kg	114 min
500 gm	205 mmol/kg	167 min

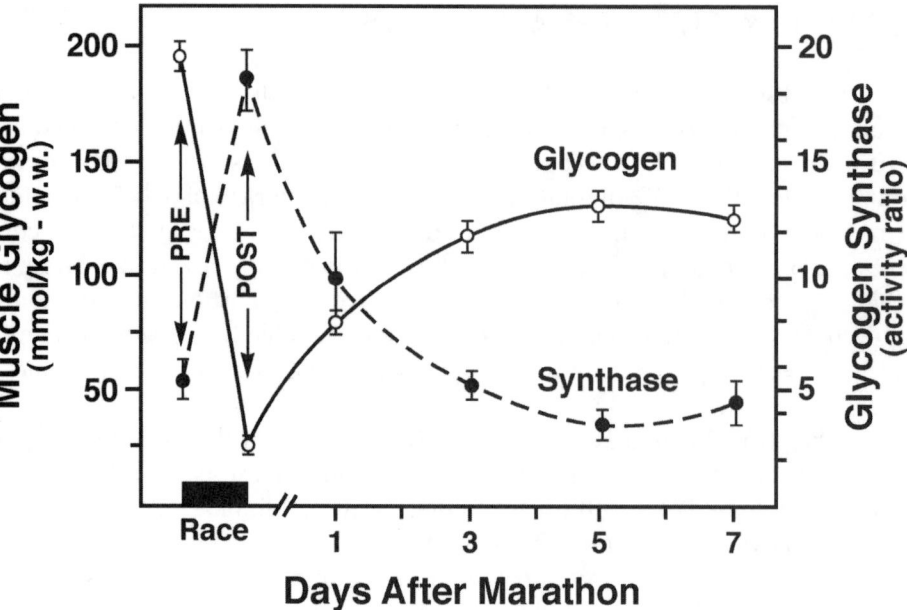

Figure 3-1. Levels of muscle glycogen and synthase activity ratios before and for seven days following the Athens, Ohio Marathon. Note that when muscle glycogen is low (post-marathon), the stimulus for glycogen storage (synthetase) is high.

mation. Even in the presence of a high glycogen synthase activity, muscle glycogen replacement is slow and incomplete unless the dietary intake is rich in carbohydrate.

Figure 3-2 demonstrates that when runners trained heavily and ate low-carbohydrate diets (40% of total calories), they had a day-to-day decline in muscle glycogen. When the same subjects ate high-carbohydrate diets (70% of total calories) of equal caloric content, muscle glycogen replacement was nearly complete within the 22 hours separating the training bouts. As you might expect, the runners perceived the training as much less difficult when they ate the high-carbohydrate diet. On the other hand, few of the runners could complete the full two hours of effort on the third day of the low-carbohydrate diet when muscle glycogen was very low.

In that study the subjects were required to consume calories that equaled their calculated total daily expenditures of approximately 4,000 kcal/day. Since many of these calories in the high-carbohydrate diet came from such complex carbohydrates as pasta, bread, and potatoes, the volume of food required was usually more than the runners wished to eat.

When subjects eat only as much food as they desire, *ad labium,* they often underestimate their caloric needs and fail to consume enough carbohydrate to compensate for that used during training or competition. This discrepancy between glycogen use and carbohydrate intake may explain, in part, why some runners become chronically fatigued and need 48 hours or longer to completely restore muscle glycogen. Runners who train exhaustively on successive days must

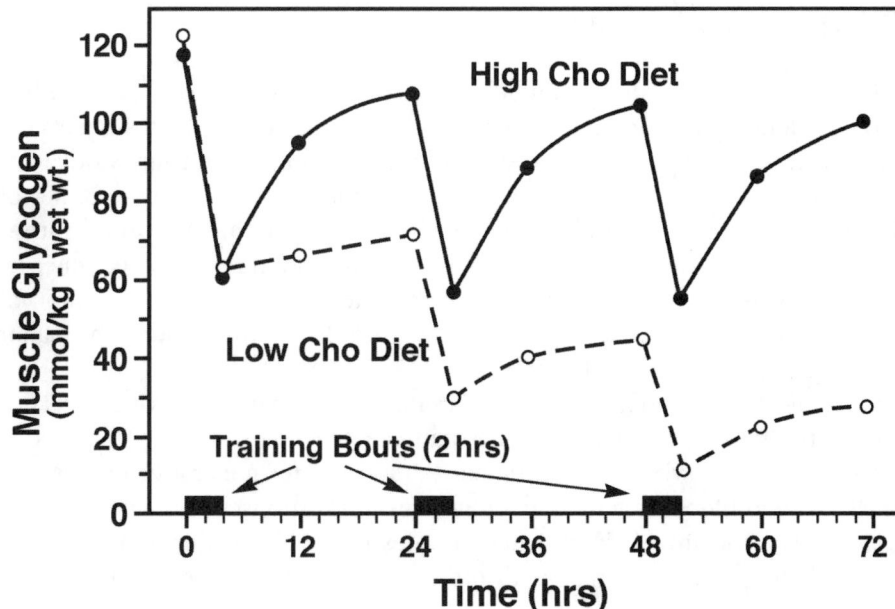

Figure 3-2. *Muscle glycogen content of the vastus lateralis (thigh) during three successive days of heavy training with diets and caloric compositions of 40% carbohydrate (low CHO) and 70% carbohydrate (high CHO).*

consume a diet rich in carbohydrates to reduce the heavy, tired feeling associated with a deficit in muscle glycogen.

So, that might be part of the explanation for why we experience "good days and bad days." If your energy supply is low, some of the muscle fibers you most frequently call on to generate the force for running may fatigue easily or may not develop the expected tension you expect. Consequently, you may sense that it takes more effort to run at a given pace than when you are rested and have plenty of muscle glycogen.

ANOTHER SIDE TO CARBOHYDRATE RICH DIETS

Is there a down-side to eating a diet rich in carbohydrates? Although athletes need supplemental carbohydrates during intense training periods, untrained individuals who consume excessive carbohydrates under normal conditions may elevate their plasma triglyceride levels, which has been associated with a high risk of heart disease. In the endurance runner, supplemental carbohydrates restore muscle and liver glycogen rather than form blood fats.

Marathoners have quite low blood triglycerides, averaging less than 50 mg/100ml of blood, compared to non-marathoners of a similar age, whose blood triglycerides may range from 80 to 120 mg/100 ml of blood. Of course, there are some individuals who may become hypertriglyceridemic (very high blood triglycerides) after high carbohydrate and/or fat diets.

TYPES OF CARBOHYDRATES

The type of carbohydrate, simple or complex, also has a bearing on the formation of blood cholesterol and other fat-related molecules. When subjects eat simple sugars such as glucose or sucrose, blood cholesterol and triglyceride concentrations increase more than they do when subjects eat the same number of calories in the form of starch. Since the simple sugars are absorbed rather quickly, their ingestion results in hyperglycemia, a sudden rise in blood glucose, which overloads the cells' energy-producing system, favoring the formation of blood fats and cholesterol. Complex carbohydrates like starch produce a smaller rise in blood glucose and cholesterol.

Since most observations have been limited to relatively inactive subjects, it is speculative to suggest that the same patterns will occur among trained distance runners. Nevertheless, endurance-trained athletes generally demonstrate a smaller rise in blood glucose and a lower insulin response even when sucrose (table sugar)is consumed. Endurance athletes divert the majority of carbohydrate foods to glycogen storage with little disturbance in their blood lipid (fat and cholesterol) levels.

In light of the differences in simple and complex carbohydrates, you might anticipate differences in the rate and quantity of glycogen deposited in the muscles following diets rich in either glucose or starch. Tests of this theory, however, are inconclusive. We studied six men who were fed diets principally composed of either simple sugars (i.e., glucose) or starches (70% of calories from pasta) for two days following exhaustive exercise. No significant difference in muscle glycogen formation was found between the two diets, although there was a trend toward greater glycogen storage when the runners consumed starch. Subsequent studies, on the other hand, have shown that simple carbohydrates promote glycogen storage to a greater extent than complex carbohydrates. So, when you want to restore your muscle and liver glycogen levels after a hard race or training run, it doesn't seem to make much difference whether you eat simple or complex carbohydrates. A large pasta meal may be just as effective as drinking a sugar or sports drink. The key to glycogen recovery is the amount of carbohydrate you consume, and the amount of time that it takes to recover. Both of these points will be discussed later.

DIET BEFORE COMPETITION

In the preceding discussion we have shown that different diets can markedly influence muscle glycogen stores and that endurance performance depends in part on the glycogen content at the onset of exercise. Based on muscle biopsy studies in the mid-1960s, a plan was formed to help runners store the maximum amount of glycogen possible, a process known as "**glycogen loading**."

The plan proposed that runners prepare for endurance competition by completing an exhaustive training run seven days before the event. For the following three days, they were instructed to eat a rich fat and protein diet to elevate glycogen synthase. In the days leading up to the competition the runner's diet was altered to contain extremely rich carbohydrates. The intensity and volume of training during the six-day period was markedly reduced to prevent additional combustion of muscle glycogen and to maximize liver and muscle glycogen reserves.

While this regimen has been shown to elevate muscle glycogen to twice the normal level, it is somewhat impractical for runners. During the three days of low carbohydrate intake, runners generally find it difficult to do even light running, are unable to perform mental tasks, are irritable, and show the usual signs of low blood sugar. In addition, exhaustive "depletion" runs performed seven days before the competition are of little training value, and may impair glycogen storage rather than enhance it. These runs also expose the runners to possible injury or overtraining when they are already susceptible to breakdown.

Considering these limitations, we have proposed that the "depletion run" and low carbohydrate aspects of this regimen be eliminated, and that the runner simply reduce the training intensity and eat a normal mixed diet containing 55% of its calories from carbohydrates, until the final three days before the competition. In the 48 to 72 hours before the race, training should be reduced to a daily warm-up of one to three easy miles, and consume a rich carbohydrate diet. Following this plan, glycogen is elevated to 200 mmol/kg of muscle, a level equal to that attained with the more elaborate Scandinavian regimen.

Diet also plays an important role in preparing the liver for the demands of distance running. Studies have shown that liver glycogen stores will decrease rapidly when an individual is deprived of carbohydrates for only 24 hours, even when at rest. As a result of strenuous exercise lasting 60 minutes, liver glycogen was found to decrease from 244 to 111 mmol/kg of muscle, a 55% reduction. In combination with a low carbohydrate diet, hard training may empty the liver glycogen stores. A single carbohydrate meal, however, will quickly restore liver glycogen to normal. Clearly, a rich carbohydrate diet in the days preceding competition will insure a large liver glycogen reserve and minimize the risk of hypoglycemia during the race.

Since water (H_2O) is stored as part of the glycogen molecule (roughly 2.6 gm of H_2O for each gm of glycogen), an increase or decrease in tissue glycogen generally produces a change in body weight of from one to three pounds. One of the most practical ways to monitor your muscle-liver glycogen stores is to note your early morning weight, recorded immediately after rising and emptying your bladder and before eating breakfast. Any sudden drop in weight may reflect a failure to replace glycogen, or a deficit in body water, or both.

PRE-RACE FOODS

The pre-competition meal should be taken three to four hours before the race and contain few fats and proteins since they digest slowly and do not provide fuels that are readily used during the race. One possible choice for this pre-race feeding might be cereal, toast, and juice since it digests quickly and will leave a minimum of residue in the stomach.

To this point, it would appear that carbohydrates can do no harm; they replace muscle and liver glycogen, maintain blood glucose, and provide the primary fuel for endurance performance. The one time that the runner should not consume carbohydrates is during the final 60-90 minutes before a long hard run. As early as 1939, studies showed that in some individuals such feedings temporarily elevate blood glucose and insulin. Since insulin transports glucose out of the blood and into the body tissues, elevated blood insulin at the beginning of exercise may result in a rapid uptake of glucose by the muscles with a sudden drop in the sugar content of the blood.

Blood glucose declines rapidly within the first 15 minutes of exercise when sugar is consumed 45 minutes before exercise (Figure 3-3). Elevated blood glucose and insulin levels at the onset of exercise also tend to suppress the liver's normal release of glucose, making it difficult for the body to quickly readjust the glucose after it has fallen to the low levels seen at 15 to 45 minutes of exercise. Although the runners seldom show their symptoms of low blood sugar, they use greater amounts of muscle glycogen and become exhausted earlier as a result of the pre-exercise sugar feeding. The key here is to ingest a light carbohydrate meal roughly two hours or more before exercise so that blood insulin and glucose have adequate time to return to normal levels.

Since the muscle and liver glycogen stores are limited, encouraging the muscles to use fat in the form of free fatty acids (FFA) as an alternative fuel could reduce the threat of exhaustion. Unfortunately, eating fat does not stimulate the muscles to burn fat. Fatty foods only tend to elevate plasma triglycerides, complex fat molecules that must be broken down to free fatty acids before they can be used to produce energy.

Aside from endurance training, the only predictable way to increase free fatty acids used is to elevate their concentration in blood using a controlled regimen of fat feedings followed by the injection of heparin, an anticoagulant. Laboratory studies have demonstrated that when the blood levels of free fatty acids are elevated in this way, exercising muscles tend to use more fat and spare their glycogen reserves. The amount of glycogen used during 30 minutes of treadmill running was reduced by 40% when the blood free fatty acids were first elevated

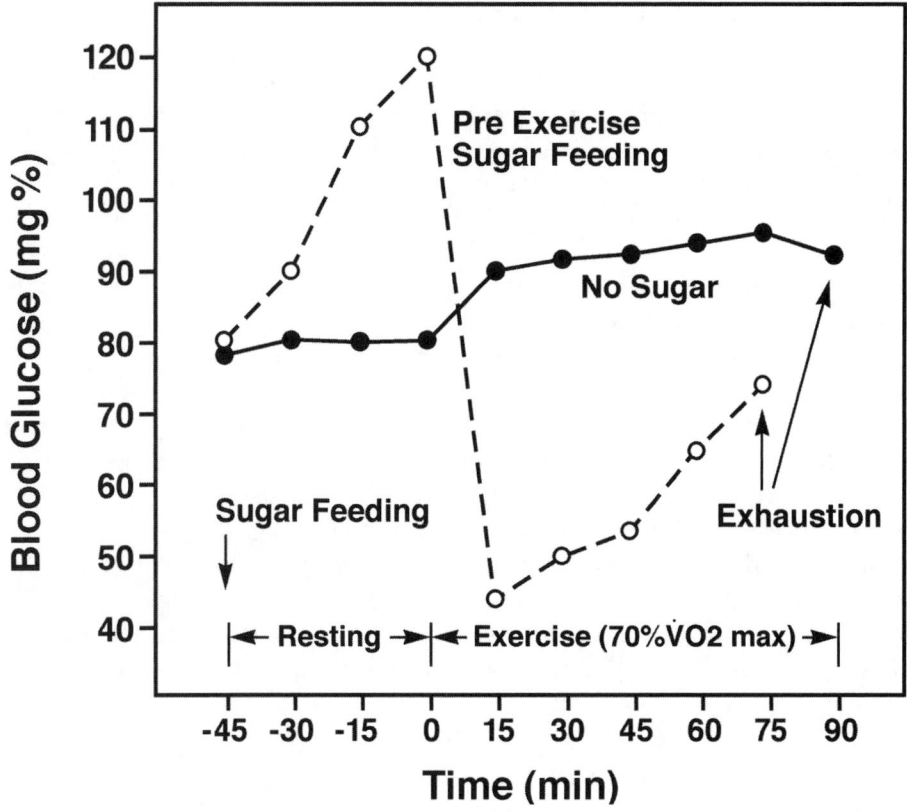

Figure **3-3.** *Effects of feeding 70 grams of glucose, taken 45 min before the onset of exercise, on blood glucose during a 90 min treadmill run.*

using the fat meal and heparin. Obviously, this point is of little value to the runner, since the use of heparin is illegal and may expose the runner to a major health risk and/or uncontrolled bleeding.

Dietary attempts to elevate plasma free fatty acids have generally been unsuccessful. Some foods that contain caffeine, a stimulant to the nervous system, appear to promote fat use and improve performance in prolonged, exhaustive exercise when consumed an hour before exercise. Caffeine ingestion of four to five mg/kg body weight lessens the subjective feelings of effort during the exercise, which is similar to the effect of amphetamines. It should be noted that international rules prohibit the use of caffeine to enhance endurance performance. Plus, 20% of the individuals tested experienced a negative reaction (e.g. headaches) to caffeine, with no improvements in performance.

Despite the potential performance advantages offered by drinking tea or coffee, the ethical use of these items is questionable since they offer an unnatural advantage. Though international governing bodies like the International Olympic Committee have attempted to ban the use of such stimulants, policing their use is difficult and impractical.

NUTRIENTS DURING DISTANCE RUNNING

Studies conducted early in this century noted the occurrence of low blood glucose during exhaustive long-distance running and cycling. Although it seems reasonable to assume that such a decrease in blood glucose might contribute to the feeling of fatigue, recent studies have suggested that hypoglycemia may not be directly to blame. In those studies, 142 minutes of exhaustive exercise dropped blood glucose from normal levels of 5.0 mmol/liter of blood to 2.5 mmoles in 30 to 40% of the subjects, the intake of glucose during exercise did not consistently delay exhaustion.

In contrast, other studies have noted improvements in performance when the subjects were given carbohydrate feedings during exercise lasting one to four hours. Although none of these studies noticed any differences in performance during the early phase of the exercise when carbohydrates were given, the subjects were able to perform better over the final stage of the experiments. We recently observed that repeated carbohydrate feedings during four hours of cycling reduced muscle glycogen depletion and improved the ability to sprint at the end of the activity. Though it has been suggested that sugar feedings during exercise might prevent the depletion of muscle glycogen, this point is debatable. It has been argued that elevating blood glucose via carbohydrate feedings enables the muscles to obtain more of their energy from the available glucose, lowering the demands placed on muscle glycogen. The runner can, therefore, go longer before the muscle glycogen stores become exhausted.

One may wonder why carbohydrate feedings during exercise do not produce the same hypoglycemic effects observed with the pre-exercise feedings. As you can see in Figure 3-4, sugar feedings given during exercise result in a smaller rise in blood glucose, lessening the threat of an over-reaction and a sudden drop in blood glucose. The cause for this finer control on blood glucose during exercise may be related to the fact that the muscle fibers become more permeable, allowing glucose to enter the muscle with the aid of less insulin. As a result, less insulin is released from the pancreas and the rise in blood glucose is smaller. Feedings before and during exercise may also help to replenish the liver glycogen reserves, thereby making the maintenance of blood sugar more constant.

The only complication associated with sugar feedings during distance running is a delay in absorption. Before sugar solutions can be absorbed into the blood, they must pass through the stomach and into the small intestine. Since most carbohydrate solutions are held in the stomach for a short period, the first traces of any sugar solution do not appear in the blood for five to seven minutes after consumption. The delay is caused by the stomach's attempts to dilute the solution and offer the intestine fluids that can be rapidly absorbed. As we will discuss later in this chapter, there are a number of factors to consider when selecting a carbohydrate drink during distance running.

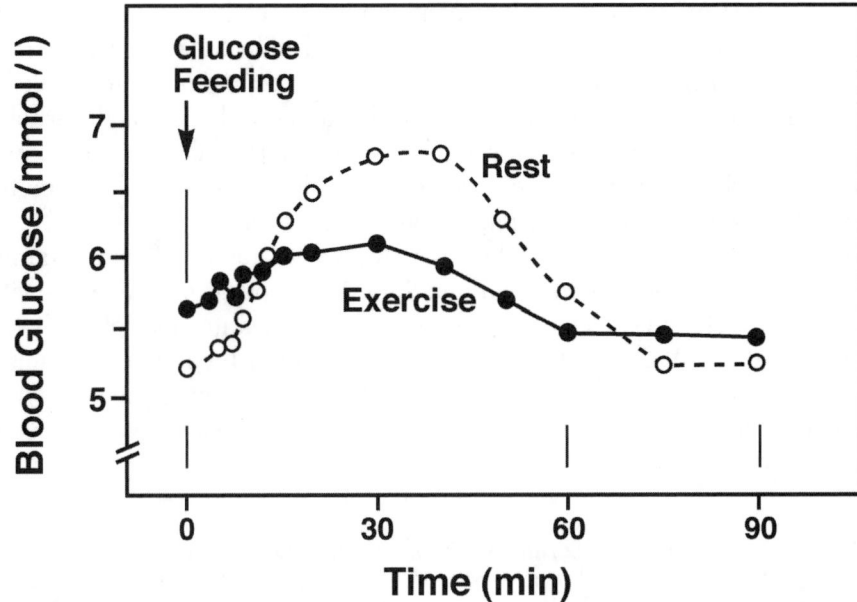

Figure 3-4. *Changes in blood glucose following a sugar feeding of 70 grams under resting and exercising conditions. Note the smaller rise in glucose when the subjects were running.*

EATING HABITS OF RUNNERS

Although we have learned a great deal from our research regarding the nutritional needs of runners before, during, and even after exercise, we know little about what they actually eat. To gain a little insight into their real practices, we had a group of runners record everything they ate and drank over a three-day period. Information was obtained in training periods and during the three days before a marathon. Our sample included athletes with a broad range of abilities, from a 2 h: 9 min marathoner, to others with personal records of nearly four hours. Their training mileages varied from a high of 19 to a low of 3 miles per day, at training paces ranging from 6 to 13 minutes per mile.

We analyzed each respondent's diet to determine the percentages of fats, proteins, and carbohydrates consumed. We also looked at whether the diets provided the Recommended Daily Allowance (RDA) of vitamins and minerals. Finally, efforts were made to match the number of calories consumed with calories used each day.

We found that there was little difference between what elite and average runners ate. Diet could not be used as a single predictor of performance. Although specific items in the diets varied—from pork chops to pasta, from collard greens to candy bars—differences blurred over a period of days when food was analyzed for its percentages of fat, proteins, and carbohydrates, or amounts of vitamins and minerals. One interesting finding was how closely runners came to meeting the RDA, the standard considered necessary for good health.

The runners we studied ate diets containing 50% carbohydrates, 36% fats, and 14% proteins. In light of the need for a high carbohydrate diet when training for distance running, we might at first consider the carbohydrate intake of these runners to be low. These runners actually ate more then enough carbohydrate to meet the energy needed for training. Since their total calorie intake was nearly 50% higher than would be expected for individuals of similar size (145 pounds), their total carbohydrate intake was well above average (Table 3-2).

We also wanted to ascertain that their diets contained sufficient vitamins and minerals to guarantee good health and maximum performance. Some vitamins are essential in the production of energy and the maintenance of the body's normal operation. Without vitamins such as the vitamin B complex, one might have trouble converting carbohydrates into ATP or forming glycogen. These runners consumed adequate vitamins and minerals to at least equal the RDA,

TABLE 3-2. A comparison of 22 runners' diets with the RDA (Recommended Daily Allowance) guidelines. Figures shown in parantheses represent estimates of the average values in the American diet, which may or may not be healthy. Even where the figure is low (as with folic acid and vitamin E), that does not necessarily suggest a deficiency since the RDA is somewhat arbitrary with a large safety factor included in their estimate.

Diet Composition	Runner's Average	RDA
Calories (kcal/day)	3,012	(2,000)
Carbohydrate (gm)	375	(250)
Protein (gm)	112	(70)
Saturated fats (gm)	42	(26)
Unsaturated fats (gm)	64	(54)
Total fat (gm)	122	(66–100)
Cholesterol (mg)	377	(300)
Fiber (gm)	7	(3–6)
Vitamin A (IU)	10,814	5,000
Vitamin B_1 (mg)	1.9	1.3
Vitamin B_2 (mg)	2.5	1.6
Vitamin B_6 (mg)	2.2	2
Vitamin B_{12} (ug)	3.8	3
Folic acid (mg)	0.23	0.4
Niacin (mg)	27.3	16
Pantothenic acid (mg)	5.3	7.5
Vitamin C (mg)	205	55
Vitamin E (mg)	5.2	14
Iron (mg)	25	14
Potassium (gm)	4.3	2.5
Calcium (gm)	1.3	1.0
Magnesium (gm)	0.4	0.3
Phosphorus (gm)	2.0	1.0
Sodium (gm)	2.6	(6.0)

which contains a built-in cushion. Unless a runner's vitamin intake falls well below the RDA for an extended period, no effects on performance would be expected. Though diets rich in simple carbohydrates tend to be deficient in some of the B complex vitamins, only two runners appeared to consume too little vitamin B_{12}.

Although some experts have suggested that we need 1,000 mg of vitamin C per day, the RDA is only 60, well below that consumed by the runners in our survey. Most of the runners did not use vitamin supplements, contrary to some recent surveys about the habits of runners. Our participants also obtained more than adequate amounts of minerals, including iron, as well as ample fiber, another item associated with good health.

In the last three days before a marathon, our subjects changed both their training and eating habits. Where previously they had averaged 8.5 miles per day, they reduced their daily mileage to 2.3. In an apparent attempt to load their muscles with glycogen, the runners increased their daily caloric intake from 3,012 kilocalories during training to a pre-marathon average of 3,730. Several ate more than 5,000 kilocalories, nearly twice their rate of caloric expenditure during that period.

Will eating excessively during the final days before a race cause you to gain unwanted fat? It might be argued that since these marathoners had reduced their training, they were gaining a daily surplus of 1,204 kcal. Theoretically this might have resulted in the storage of one extra pound of unnecessary fat (3,600 kilocalories equals one pound of fat). From the standpoint of marathon performance, however, it is probably better to eat a bit too much food, principally carbohydrates, than to risk not being fully loaded with muscle and liver glycogen.

FLUID BALANCE

The ability to lose body heat during distance running depends, for the most part, on the formation and evaporation of sweat. The amount of sweat lost during exercise is somewhat proportional to your running pace, body size, and the heat stress imposed by the environment. Running in warm weather may evoke sweat losses in excess of two quarts per hour. Despite efforts to drink fluids during a marathon, sweating and the loss of water in the air we breathe may reduce body water content by 13 to 14%.

Studies have shown that dehydrated runners are quite intolerant of exercise and heat stress. Distance runners are forced to slow their pace by 2% for each percentage of loss in body weight due to dehydration. In addition, both heart rate and body temperature are elevated during exercise when runners are dehydrated more than 2% of their body weight.

The impact of dehydration on the cardiovascular system is quite predictable. Plasma volume is lost and the ability to provide adequate blood flow to the skin and muscle is reduced. In this situation, it is common for runners to collapse, showing the usual symptoms of heat exhaustion. It is difficult to understand how some athletes tolerate several hours of hard running in warm weather. In addition to the body water lost during heavy sweating, many essential nutrients are also lost. The following discussion will examine the effects of heavy sweating on body water and the mineral composition of body tissues.

Human sweat has been described as a "filtrate of plasma," since it contains many of the items present in the water portion of blood, including sodium chloride, potassium, magnesium, and calcium. However, even though sweat tastes salty, it actually contains far fewer minerals than other body fluids. Sweat is considered hypotonic, meaning it is a very dilute (containing mostly water) version of body fluids.

Sodium and chloride are the ions primarily responsible for maintaining the water content of the blood. The concentrations of these minerals in sweat are roughly one third those found in plasma and five times those found in muscle (Table 3-3). Their concentration in sweat may vary markedly between individuals and is influenced by the rate of sweating and the runner's state of prior exposure to heat stress (i.e., heat acclimation).

At the high rates of sweating reported during distance running, sweat contains relatively high levels of sodium and chloride, but little potassium, calcium, and magnesium. A sweat loss of nearly nine pounds, representing a 5.8% reduction in body weight, resulted in sodium, potassium, chloride, and magnesium losses of roughly 155, 16, 137, and 13 mEq, respectively. Based on estimates of the runner's body mineral contents, these losses would be expected to lower the body's sodium and chloride content by roughly 5 to 7%. At the same time, total body levels of potassium and magnesium, two ions principally confined to the inside of the cells, decreased by less than 1.2%.

The other major source of mineral loss is through the production of urine. In addition to clearing the blood of cellular waste products, the kidneys also control the body's water and electrolyte content. Under normal conditions, kidneys excrete about 1.7 ounces of water per hour. During exercise, however, blood flow to the kidneys decreases, and urine production drops to near zero. Consequently, electrolyte losses by this avenue are quite diminished during exercise.

TABLE 3-3. Electrolyte concentrations and osmolarity in sweat, plasma, and muscle.

	Electrolytes (mEq/liter)				Osmolality (mOsm/liter)
	Na^+	Ci^-	K^+	Mg^{++}	
SWEAT	40–60	30–50	4–5	1.5–5	80–185
PLASMA	140	101	4	1.5	302
MUSCLE	9	6	162	31	302

Na^+ = sodium; Cl^- = chloride; K^+ = potassium; Mg^{++} = magnesium
osmolality—number of particles contained in a solution

There is another facet of the kidneys' management of electrolytes. If an individual eats 250 mEq of sodium and chloride per day, normally the kidneys will excrete an equal amount of those electrolytes to keep their levels constant within the body. Heavy sweating and dehydration, however, cause the release of aldosterone, a hormone from the adrenal gland that stimulates the kidneys to reabsorb sodium and chloride.

Since the body loses more water than electrolytes during heavy sweating, the concentration of these minerals in the body fluids rises. That means that instead of showing a drop in plasma electrolyte concentrations, there is actually an increase. Although this may seem confusing, the point is that during periods of heavy sweating, the need to replace body water is greater than the need to replace electrolytes.

There are obvious benefits from drinking fluids during prolonged exercise, especially during hot weather. Drinking will minimize dehydration, lessen the rise in internal body temperature, and reduce the stress placed on the circulatory system. Warm fluids near body temperature provide some protection against overheating, but cold fluids seem to enhance body cooling. It takes some of the deep body heat to warm a cold drink to the temperature of the gut.

The fluid composition of the drink also has an effect on the rate that it empties from the stomach. Since little exchange of water occurs directly from the stomach, the fluids must pass into the intestine before entering the blood. In the intestine, absorption is rapid and unaffected by exercise, provided that the activity does not exceed 75% of the runner's $\dot{V}O_2$max. Many factors affect the rate at which the stomach will empty, including its volume, temperature, acidity, and osmolality.

Large volumes of fluid up to 600 ml (20 oz.) empty faster from the stomach than small portions. Runners, however, generally find it uncomfortable to run with a nearly full stomach, as this interferes with breathing. Drinking three to six ounces at 10 to 15 minute intervals tends to minimize this effect. We have, however, observed dramatically different rates of stomach-emptying among individual runners. The suggestions offered here are based on averages and may not be appropriate you. Only trial and error will determine what works best for you.

Cold drinks have been found to empty more rapidly from the stomach than warm fluids. Although fluids at refrigerator temperatures of 38 to 40° F may reduce the temperature of the stomach from 99 to 40° F, they do not appear to cause stomach cramps. Such stomach distress occurs more often when the volume of the drink is unusually large. Cold fluids also may upset the normal electrical activity of the heart, threatening the health of the runner. It is true that some electrocardiographic changes have been reported in a few individuals following the ingestion of ice-cold drinks (33 to 35° F), but the medical significance of these changes has not been established. It seems that drinking cold fluids during distance running poses no threat to a normal heart.

Another factor known to regulate the rate at which the stomach empties is the drink's osmolality, the number of dissolved substances in the solution. Drink osmolality above 200 mOsm per liter tend move out of the stomach more slowly than those below that level. The addition of electrolytes and other ingredients that raise the osmolality slows the rate of water replacement. Since dehydration is the primary concern during hot weather running, water seems to be the preferred fluid. Under less stressful conditions where overheating and large sweat losses are not as threatening, runners might use liquid feedings to supplement their carbohydrate supplies.

A number of "sports drinks", containing carbohydrates, are currently on the market and grossing more than $100 million each year. Unfortunately, many of the claims used to sell these drinks are based on misinterpreted and often inaccurate information. Electrolytes, for example, have long been touted as important ingredients in sports drinks. But research has shown that such claims are unfounded. A single meal adequately replaces the electrolytes lost during exercise. The body needs water to bring its concentration of the electrolytes back into balance. While the importance of minerals such as sodium, potassium, and magnesium should not be underestimated, blood and muscle biopsy studies have shown that heavy sweating has little or no effect on water and electrolyte concentrations in body fluids.

One might wonder if the intake of too much water could over dilute the blood electrolytes, leading to a body concentration deficit. We originally thought this was highly unlikely. But, experience in recent years of reported cases of hyponatremia (low blood sodium) after marathons and ultra-marathon races, has raised the suspicion that some runners may be drinking far in excess of their sweat losses. Runners who have experienced severe hyponatremia (blood sodium values 10 to 20% below normal) may lapse into a coma, convulse, and in some cases die from this electrolyte imbalance. Although the precise cause of this condition is not fully understood, there is some evidence to suggest that runners who take 4 hours or more to complete a marathon may be at greater risk. Reports have surfaced which indicate that these individuals also drink large quantities of fluids, usually water, during and after the race. Under normal conditions the kidneys would be expected to unload any excess water, but that does not appear to be the case among runners who become hyponatremic. The excessive amounts of fluid they consumed appeared to cause a dilution of blood sodium, and subsequent hyponatremia. The risk of becoming hyponatremic appears to be low, but should not be ignored.

So, how do you keep from becoming a victim of hyponatremia? In most cases, the problem appears to occur because the runners continue to drink far in excess of their thirst after the race. One approach would be to weigh yourself before and immediately after the race. If your body weight at the finish is within a couple of pounds of the pre-race level, then you don't need any fluids, whether you are thirsty or not. In any event, your body weight should not be above the pre-race level.

FLUID INTAKE DURING THE RACE

Should the fluids consumed during the race contain minerals (i.e., sodium, potassium, etc.)? Under normal conditions distance runners who lose six to nine pounds of sweat and drink nearly a half-gallon of water will retain normal plasma sodium, chloride, and potassium concentrations. In several studies, marathoners and ultra-marathoners who ran 15 to 25 miles per day in warm weather and did not season their food, experienced no electrolyte deficiencies. Even when we fed test subjects only 30% as much potassium as they normally consumed and made them dehydrate by losing seven to eight pounds of sweat every day for eight days, body electrolytes remained unchanged. Though it can be argued that water is as effective as an electrolyte solution (e.g., sports drinks)in maintaining hydration, there may be a small advantage in using drinks that provide some minerals and nutrients.

There is evidence to support putting some carbohydrates in sports drinks, including several types of sugar. Structurally, the simplest forms of sugar are the monosaccharide (i.e., glucose, and fructose). While even small amounts of glucose tend to slow the emptying of the stomach, adding fructose can be used without inhibiting the stomach's action. Aside from this, there is little difference whether the carbohydrate in the drink is glucose or fructose, since both take five to seven minutes before they first appear in the blood.

In our early studies, we suggested that the runner's drink should have less than 2.5 grams of sugar per 100 milliliters of water to speed its removal from the stomach. Unfortunately, this small amount of carbohydrate contributes little to your energy supply. Even if you drank 200 ml of a drink every 15 minutes during a long run, you might only take in 20 grams of carbohydrate per hour. Our recent studies suggest that to improve performance with the aid of a carbohydrate drink, the runner must consume at least 50 grams of sugar per hour.

Most of the sports drinks on the market contain only about 0.6 grams of carbohydrate per ounce. A runner would have to drink a half-gallon of these drinks every hour to get enough carbohydrates to do any good. Since we know that most runners drink only nine to 15 ounces per hour during long runs, it would take a drink containing 3.8 grams of carbohydrate per ounce to be of any value. Such a rich mixture, however, might be delayed in the stomach, draw water from the stomach's lining, and cause an uncomfortable feeling of fullness.

Recent technological advances in the manufacture of carbohydrates have made it possible to combine many glucose molecules into one large molecule called a "glucose polymer." Using it, a drink does not have such a negative effect on the stomach and replaces both water and carbohydrates. The best mixture of carbohydrates for the runner's drink would be one containing small amounts of fructose and a sizeable quantity of the glucose polymer.

Finally, runners will not drink something that does not taste good. Since we all have different taste preferences, it is difficult to find one solution that is palatable for everyone. To confuse the issue even further, what tastes good before and after a long, hot run will not necessarily taste good during the race. We conducted a series of taste tests before and after a 60 minute run to determine what type of drinks runners preferred. These studies demonstrated that most of the 50 subjects chose a drink with a relatively light flavor which did not have a strong aftertaste. In this regard, nearly all of the commercial sports drinks failed.

So what should the runner drink during the training and competition? Under the extreme stress of hot weather, water is the primary need and the preferred drink. It empties from the stomach with minimal delay, is easy to obtain, and reduces the dehydration associated with heavy sweating. Under cooler conditions, a carbohydrate drink will provide the lift needed for peak performance in events lasting an hour or longer.

It is important to realize that human thirst is a poor indicator of the body's water and electrolyte balance. No matter how efficiently the kidneys do their job, body fluid balance depends on a strong thirst sensation to stimulate fluid intake. Unfortunately, a human's drive to replace body fluids is far less effective than that seen in other animals. Burros, for example, will replace a 40-pound body water loss in five to six minutes of continuous drinking, whereas humans who sweat away six to eight pounds are satisfied after drinking only a few ounces of fluid. If the runner's thirst is used as the only gauge of water need, it would take 12 to 24 hours to replace such a sweat loss.

SPECIAL DIETS AND SUPPLEMENTS

Athletes are always looking for an edge, something that will give them an advantage. Since the difference between winning and losing can often be measured in fractions of a second, no athlete wants to feel that he or she did not try everything possible to achieve a best performance. Manipulating the diet and taking extra quantities of various vitamins and minerals seem to be relatively harmless methods to make the body work its best. But do these efforts really help?

Vitamins are organic substances necessary for growth and cellular function. Though some vitamins can be produced in small quantities in the body and others stored in the body fat, most must be consumed in the diet (Table 3-4). Vitamins C and B complex, for example, are water soluble, cannot be stored, and must be constantly replenished by the diet. The fat-soluble vitamins (A, D, E, and K) are stored in the liver and fatty tissue of the body and can accumulate during a period of excess intake for use at times when they may not be readily available.

Unfortunately, there is no way to judge vitamin levels, unless a person has a deficiency. Only then do rather unpleasant symptoms appear. The characteristic sores and loss of vision associated with a deficiency in vitamin B_2 (riboflavin), for

TABLE 3-4. Dietary sources, functions, and daily requirements of selected vitamins for adults.

Vitamin	Recommended Daily Intake (I.U.)			Source	Function	Symptoms of Deficiency
	Non-Athlete	Strength Athlete	Endurance Athlete			
A (I.U.)	5,000	10,000	10,000	Liver, Egg Yolk, Milk	Prevents Eye and Skin Disorders	Night Blindness
B_1 (mg)	1.4	4.6	6–10	Meat, Grains, Milk	Energy Metabolism	Beriberi
B_2 (mg)	1.6	3.0	4.0	Milk, Fish, Meat, Green Vegetables	Energy Metabolism	Mouth & Lip Lesions, Loss of Vision
B_6 (mg)	2.0	2.0	2.0	Bananas, Spinach, Greens	Protein & Glycogen Metabolism	Anemia and Convulsions
Niacin (mg)	18	25	35	Peanut Butter, Greens, Fish	Fatty Acid Metabolism	Low Energy Production
B_{12} (ug)	5	10	10	Animal Foods	Energy Metabolism, nervous system function	Anemia, Muscular Weakness
Folic Acid (mg)	0.4	0.4	0.4	Greens, Mushrooms, Liver	Blood Cell Production	Anemia
C (mg)	60	100–200	100–200	Citrus Fruits, Tomatoes	Growth	Scurvy
D (I.U.)	400	400	400	Sunlight, Fish, Eggs	Absorption of Calcium	Rickets
E (I.U.)	20	40	60	Vegetable Oils, Greens	Antioxidant (7)	Unknown

example, are rare in our society. Treatment with foods and tablets containing the essential vitamins generally eliminates the symptoms.

The earlier discussion regarding our survey of runners' diets demonstrated that, on the average, the intake of vitamins was equal to or greater than the RDA. Individually, however, a number of the runners were eating diets containing less than the RDA for vitamins B_6, B_{12}, pantothenic acid, and folic acid. When we consider that the levels needed of these vitamins vary in proportion to the number of calories consumed in the diet, things looked even worse. Some of the runners were taking in less than 50% of the recommended amount of these vitamins, based on the number of calories they were eating. One explanation for the low levels may be that some of the runners were vegetarians or ate diets low in such animal products as meats, cheese, milk, and eggs, which are the principal sources of B_6, B_{12}, and pantothenic acid.

Even though some runners consumed low levels of certain B vitamins, none of the runners exhibited any symptoms of vitamin B deficiencies, such as anemia or unusual fatigue. Despite such assurances, some of the runners were taking vitamin supplements, containing two to five times the amounts recommended by the RDA (Recommended Daily Allowance).

Over the past 40 years a variety of attempts have been made to resolve the question of whether vitamins taken in doses greater than the RDA will enhance performance and produce better health. To state that the research findings showed no benefits of vitamin supplementation would be inaccurate and somewhat misleading. There have been a number of studies that found increased endurance with enormous doses of vitamins C, E, and B complex, but there are far more studies demonstrating that vitamins in excess of the RDA will not improve performance in either strength or endurance activities. Experts generally agree that popping vitamins will not make up for a lack of talent or training or give one an edge over the competition.

As a matter of fact, too much of a good thing can be harmful. Extremely large doses of vitamins A and D may produce some undesirable effects. Large overdoses of vitamin A, for example, may cause a loss of appetite, loss of hair, enlargement of the liver and spleen, swelling over the long bones, and general irritability—scarcely ideal conditions for a good distance runner. We have never seen these symptoms, however, even in athletes taking two to three times the RDA for these vitamins.

All in all, it appears that the RDA values for the various vitamins are about optimal for normal body operations, though possibly on the conservative side. Certainly, there is no convincing evidence to prove that vitamin pills taken to supplement a balanced diet will improve endurance or running performance. Overdoses of vitamins may be of some value, if for some reason you wish to increase the vitamin content of your urine, since that is where most of the excess ends up. Perhaps that is why it is said that athletes have the most expensive urine in the world.

In recent years theoretical arguments have focused on the potentially negative effects of exercise on tissue damage and impairment of the body's immune system. In the process of generating energy the cells use hydrogen to produce water and free radicals, highly reactive molecules that can damage cellular components such as DNA and cell membranes. Fortunately, cells have protective mechanisms (i.e., antioxidants) to counter these potentially damaging free radicals. Having a diet with appropriate quantities of antioxidant vitamins, such as ß-carotene and vitamin E, have been suggested as essential to protect the cells against damage from these free radicals. In well-nourished runners, this probably is not an issue. Nevertheless, research continues on this issue, which may offer a better understanding of the role of vitamins in free radical protection. But, at this point it seems that much of the information and theories are more imaginable than factual.

Minerals are the second most widely used diet supplements by athletes. Since perspiration tastes salty, many runners fear a large loss of body salts during periods of heavy sweating. Actually, as we have pointed out, sweat is quite dilute when compared to other body fluids. There is, however, a wide individual variation in the quantity of minerals lost in sweat. Nevertheless, we have noted that fewer electrolytes are lost in the sweat of highly trained and heat-acclimatized runners than in untrained individuals. It is fair to state that the mineral content of a balanced diet can easily off-set the electrolytes lost in sweat. It is interesting to note that individuals who eat a low-salt diet excrete sweat that is low in sodium. Apparently the body adjusts the electrolyte content of sweat to keep pace with dietary intake. Even without mineral supplements, the body can get all it needs from the natural minerals in food.

Iron is an essential component of hemoglobin, the oxygen-carrying component of blood, and of myoglobin, the oxygen-transporting pigment of muscle. Since iron deficiency anemia is known to impair endurance performance, it is important to distinguish between true anemia and the plasma volume dilution associated with repeated days of training in warm weather. Training tends to increase the volume of plasma more than the number of red blood cells, producing a drop in hemoglobin concentration with no apparent effect on oxygen transport or endurance.

Several studies have reported that between 36 and 82% of female runners are anemic or iron deficient. In light of this high frequency of iron deficiency in females, it seems logical to suggest that they include iron-rich foods in their diets. Iron supplementation should be directed by a physician, since prolonged administration of iron can cause an iron overload, a potentially serious condition.

DIETING AND EXERCISE

During the question and answer periods that often follow our lectures to distance runners, we are frequently asked, "How can a runner diet, lose weight, and train hard at the same time?" The answer is, "you can't." To lose fat the body must be forced to rely more heavily on its fat reserves for energy, while taking in little fuel. This results in a "caloric deficit" and a gradual reduction in the body's fat weight. Though a diet-exercise regimen accelerates the rate of weight loss, it fails to allow for adequate replacement of muscle and liver glycogen stores. As a result, dieting runners feel heavy, are easily fatigued, and are able to train only at a relatively slow pace and with reduced mileage.

Attempts to lose weight should be scheduled for periods when you do not intend to prepare for competition. During those periods, you can afford to put in the long, slow miles that stimulate the burning of fat. Though exercise aids in losing weight, the only way known to insure the removal of body fat is partial starvation. Too bad it isn't as easy or as enjoyable to get rid of body fat as it is to put it on!

LESSONS LEARNED

Hopefully in the preceding discussion we have made it clear that proper nutrition can play an important role in distance running performance. The key to success is the availability of carbohydrates for muscle energy, though fat serves as an alternative fuel source and contributes to the energy pool during the long, slower paced runs. The storage of muscle glycogen depends on a rich carbohydrate diet, though a complement of all the basic food groups, vitamins, and minerals are essential for peak performance. Repeated days of intense training can result in a slow recovery of muscle glycogen, leading to a chronic state of fatigue. On the other hand, periods of reduced training and diets supplemented with carbohydrate foods promote good training and the adaptations needed for improvement.

During distance events lasting for several hours, it is important to consume fluids to replace the body water lost in sweat and heavy breathing. Although a variety of minerals are lost in sweat, there is little need to replace them during exercise, since their balance in the body is easily maintained through proper nutrition and regulation by the kidneys. Inclusion of carbohydrate in the runner's drink appears to maintain blood glucose levels during long events and improve performance. Unfortunately, the addition of most forms of carbohydrate to the drink tends to slow the stomachs emptying, delaying the delivery of water and carbohydrates to the body. In hot weather, where dehydration and overheating are the major concerns, cold water is the recommended fluid to take while running. The consumption of 3.5 to 7 ounces of water every couple of miles during a long, hot run will reduce dehydration, with the least accumulation of fluid in the stomach.

Finally, runners who consume a balanced diet have little need for vitamin and mineral supplements. Though there is some evidence to show that female runners may develop an iron deficiency, it may not be accurate to generalize that all runners should supplement their diets with iron. While some runners may take less than the RDA for specific vitamins, symptoms of vitamin deficiencies have not been reported, nor have specific performance benefits been attributed to vitamin supplementation.

CLASSIC AND SUGGESTED READINGS

Bergstrom, J., L. Hermansen, E. Hultman and et al. Diet, muscle glycogen and physical performance. *Acta Physiol. Scand.*, 71:140–150, 1967.

Bunch, T. W. Blood test abnormalities in runners. *Mayo Clin. Proc.*, 55:113–117, 1980.

Claremont, A., D. Costill, W. Fink and P. Van Handel. Heat tolerance following diuretic induced dehydration. *Med. Sci. Sports*, 8:239–243, 1976.

Clement, D. B. and R. C. Asmundson. Nutritional intake and hematologic parameters in endurance runners. *Phys. Sportsmed.*, 10:37–43, 1982.

Costill, D. L., A. Bennett, G. Branam and D. Eddy. Glucose ingestion at rest and during prolonged exercise. *J. of Appl. Physiol.*, 34:764–769, 1973.

Costill, D. L. and B. Saltin. Factors limiting gastric emptying during rest and exercise. *J. Appl. Physiol.*, 37:679–683, 1974.

Costill, D. L., E. Coyle, G. Dalsky, W. Evans, W. Fink and D. Hoopes. Effects of elevated plasma FFA and insulin on muscle glycogen usage during exercise. *J. Appl. Physiol.*, 43:695–699, 1977.

Costill, D. L., G. P. Dalsky and W. J. Fink. Effects of caffeine ingestion on metabolism and exercise performance. *Med. Sci. Sports,* 10:155–158, 1978.

Costill, D. L., M. Sherman, W. Fink, C. Maresh, M. Witten and J. Miller. The role of dietary carbohydrates in muscle glycogen resynthesis after strenuous running. *Amer. Jour. of Clin. Nutr.*, 34, 1831–1836, 1981.

Costill, D. L., R. Bowers, G. Branam and et al. Muscle glycogen utilization during prolonged exercise on successive days. *J. Appl. Physiol.*, 31:834–838, 1971.

Costill, D. L., R. Cote and W. Fink. Muscle water and electrolytes following varied levels of dehydration in man. *J. Appl. Physiol.*, 40:6–11, 1976.

Costill, D. L., R. Cote and W. Fink. Dietary potassium and heavy exercise: Effects on muscle water and electrolytes. *Am. J. Clin. Nutr.*, 36:266–Z75, 1982.

Costill, D. L., R. Cote, W. Fink and P. Van Handel. Muscle water and electrolyte distribution during prolonged exercise. *Int. J. Sports Med.,* 2:130–134, 1981.

Costill, D. L., W. F. Kammer and A. Fisher. Fluid ingestion during distance running. *Arch. Environ. Health*, 21:520–525, 1970.

Costill, D. L., W. J. Fink, J. L. Ivy, L. H. Getchell and F. A. Witzmann. Lipid Metabolism in skeletal muscle of endurance-trained males and females. *Diabetes*, 28:818–822, 1979.

Coyle, E. F., J. M. Hagberg, B. F. Hurley, W. H. Martin, A. A. Ehsani and J. O. Holloszy. Carbohydrate feedings during prolonged strenuous exercise can delay fatigue. *J. Appl. Physiol.*, 55:230–235, 1983.

Fink, W. J, D. L. Costill and P. J. Van Handel. Leg muscle metabolism during exercise in the heat and cold. *Europ. J. Appl. Physiol.*, 34:183–190, 1975.

Foster, C. C., D. L. Costill and W. F. Fink. Effects of preexercise feedings on endurance performance. *Med Sci. In Sports,* 11:1–5, 1979.

Hargreaves, M., D. L. Costill, A. Coggan, W. J. Fink and I. Nishibata. Effect of carbohydrate feedings on muscle glycogen utilization and exercise performance. *Med. Sci. Sports Exer.,* 16:219–222, 1984.

Ivy, J. L., D. L. Costill, W. J. Fink and E. Maglischo. Contributions of medium and long chain triglyceride intake to energy metabolism during prolonged exercise. *Int. J. Sports Med.,* 1:15–20, 1980.

Ivy, J. L., D. L. Costill, W. J. Fink and R. W. Lower. Influence of caffeine and carbohydrate feedings on endurance performance. *Med. Sci. In Sports,* 11:6–11, 1979.

King, D. S., D. L. Costill, W. J. Fink, M. Hargreaves and R. A. Fielding. Muscle metabolism during exercise in the heat in unacclimatized and acclimatized man. *J. Appl. Physiol.* 59(5):1350–1354, 1985.

Piehl, K. Time course for refilling of glycogen stores in human muscle fibers following exercise-induced glycogen depletion. *Acta Physiol. Scand.,* 90:297–302, 1974.

Plowman, S. A. and P. C. McSwegin. The effects of iron supplementation on female cross country runners. *J. Sports Med. Phys. Fitness,* 21:407–416, 1981.

Roberts, K. M., E. G. Noble, D. B. Hayden and A. W. Taylor. The effect of simple and complex carbohydrate diets on skeletal muscle glycogen and lipoprotein lipase of marathon runners. *Clinical Physiol,* 5:41, 1985.

Sherman, W. M., D. L. Costill, W. J. Fink and J. M. Miller. Effects of exercise-diet manipulation on muscle glycogen and its subsequent utilization during performance. *Int J. Sports Med.,* 2:1–15, 1981.

Sherman, W. M., D. L. Costill, W. J. Fink, L. E. Armstrong and F. C. Hagerman. The marathon: Recovery from acute biochemical alterations. *Biochem. Exer.,* 13:312–317, 1983.

Chapter 4
Training: The Price for Success

INTRODUCTION

In its simplest form, endurance training serves as a constructive type of stress. Regular physical activity causes the body to become more tolerant of the demands of exercise so that it can run farther and faster. During each training run, the leg muscles demand that energy be supplied at a very high rate, often at 200 times the resting level. Day by day such training stress triggers the muscles and circulation to grow stronger and more capable of generating energy.

Assuming that one training program will work effectively for every runner is as logical as assuming that all runners are gifted with the same natural talents. Researchers who have evaluated different training programs are aware of the wide individual variations in endurance gains. Some runners will show very large gains in their aerobic capacities and endurance performances, whereas others may gain little from the same efforts. There are, however, some basic physiological adaptations that occur in all runners, though the magnitude of these changes may differ markedly.

Historical Note

The earliest reported training regimen for a distance runner was published by Alfred Shrubb, who held all records for distance of 2 (9 min:08.4s) to 10 miles (50 min:40.6s) in 1904. Shrubb trained twice per day, six days per week, averaging 10 miles per day.

TRANSFORMING THE MUSCLE

Repeated muscular contractions during distance running require the breakdown and rebuilding of adenosine triphosphate (ATP), which is produced and stored within the muscle fibers (see Chapter 1). Production of ATP during long, relatively slow distance runs depends almost exclusively on the availability of oxygen and the aerobic breakdown of carbohydrates and fats. Consequently, endurance training improves the mechanisms that are responsible for aerobic energy production. These improvements include: (1) better blood flow and oxygen delivery to the muscle, (2) a greater capacity for muscle fibers to produce ATP, (3) increased storage of glycogen and fat within the fibers, and (4) faster removal of waste materials produced within the fibers.

The exchange of oxygen and carbon dioxide between the blood and the muscle fiber occurs in the smallest blood vessels (capillaries) that surround each muscle cell. Training increases the number of capillaries bordering the fibers, sometimes by up to 40%. The photographs in Figure 4-1 reveal a remarkable increase in the number of capillaries in a runner before and after several months

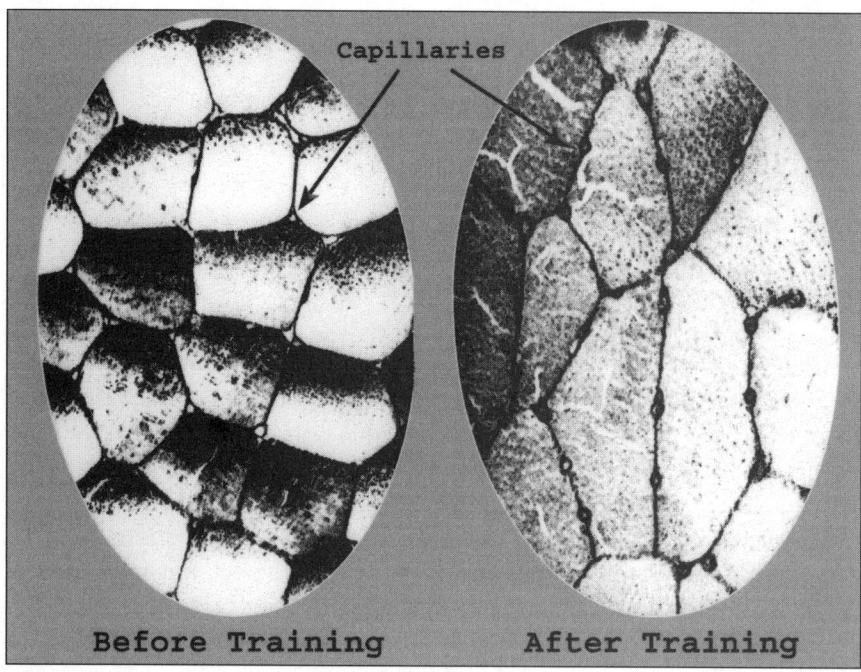

Figure 4-1. Skeletal muscle capillaries before and after several months of run training. The capillaries are cylindrical in nature and surround the perimeter of each muscle fiber. Note how many more capillaries are surrounding each fiber with training.

of endurance training. Such an increase in the number of capillaries provides for greater exchange of gases, heat, and fuels between the blood and the interior of the working muscle fiber. This maintains an advantageous environment for energy production and repeated muscle contractions.

Once oxygen is delivered to the cell membrane, it is held and transported within the fiber by myoglobin, a compound similar to hemoglobin. Myoglobin's main function is to deliver oxygen from the cell membrane to the powerhouse of the cell, the mitochondria. The myoglobin content in skeletal muscle increases significantly with endurance training. This increase in myoglobin, however, occurs only within the muscles involved in the training and does not take place in less active fibers. For example, you can't train your legs and expect your arms to gain endurance.

Aerobic energy production (ATP) is the exclusive responsibility of the mitochondria (Figure 4-2). Muscle biopsy studies have shown that there are two major changes associated with mitochondrial energy production following endurance training: an increase in the number and the size of the mitochondria. Research has shown a progressive weekly increase of approximately 5% in the number of muscle mitochondria over a 27-week period of endurance training. At the same time, the average size of the mitochondria increased from 11.5 to 15.5 microns$^2 \times 10^{-2}$, a 35% increase. These steady but gradual changes in mitochondria suggest that the structural improvements associated with endurance training may take months and perhaps years to fully develop.

RUNNING: THE ATHLETE WITHIN

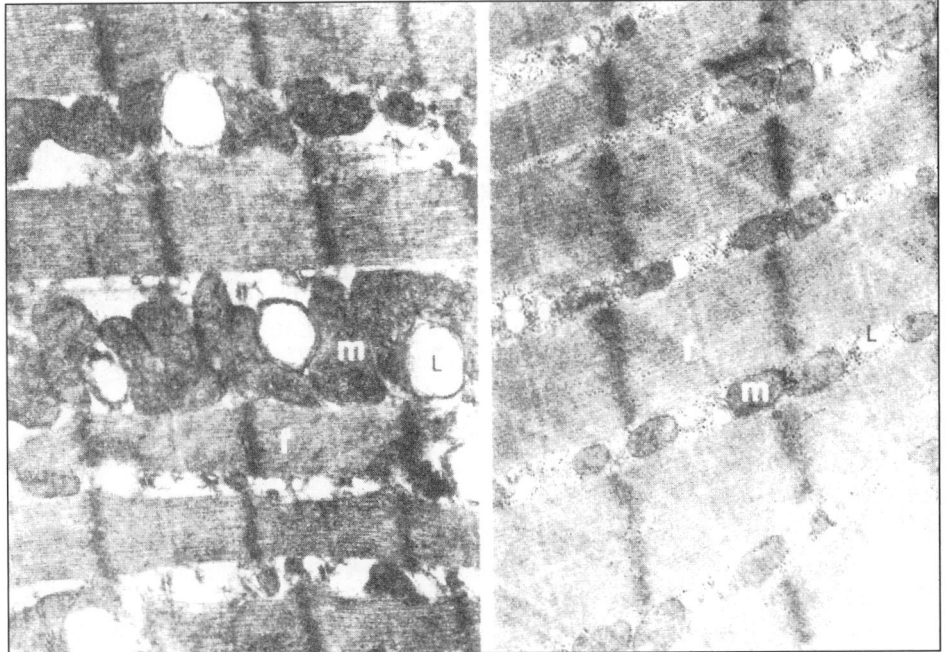

Figure 4-2. Electron micrograph looking into the leg muscle fibers of a highly trained runner (left) and an untrained man (right). Note the large number and size of the mitochondria (m) in the trained muscle. The trained fiber also has more fat (L) than the untrained muscle. Both factors provide an endurance advantage for the trained muscle.

Each mitochondria contains a large number of special proteins that speed the process of breaking-down carbohydrates and fats to produce ATP. Distance running training increases the amount of these enzymes dramatically. Table 4-1 illustrates how some of the key enzymes increase during three months of endurance training.

Special adjustments in the action of these enzymes make it possible for the endurance-trained muscle to burn fat better, lessening the demands on the limited supply of muscle glycogen. Improvements in the delivery of oxygen and its use within the muscle fiber result in a larger capacity to produce energy and to shift toward a greater reliance on fat for ATP production.

In Chapter 2 we mentioned the selective use of muscle fibers during distance running. Measurements of glycogen depletion from different muscle

TABLE 4-1. Changes in selected aerobic muscle enzymes with three months of endurance running. The enzymes shown here are SDH (succinate dehydrogenase), CPT (carintine palmityl transferase), and MDH (malate dehydrogenase). All values are mmol/kg $\times$ g $\times$ min^{-1}.

Enzyme	Before Training	After Training
SDH	8.0	21.2
CPT	1.4	2.3
MDH	126.0	225.0

fibers indicates that during long training runs and competition slow-twitch fibers are used more than the fast-twitch fibers. Only after the slow-twitch fibers begin to fatigue or the running speed is increased do the fast-twitch fibers become active.

Long, slow distance running will place most of the stress on the slow-twitch fibers, with few adaptations occurring in the fast-twitch. Incorporating more quality or speed into the training program taxes both fiber types, increasing their aerobic capacities. Likewise, when extremely long runs are incorporated into the training program, both fiber types show improvements in aerobic energy production. Fast, anaerobic running, on the other hand, produces little improvement in the muscles' aerobic capacity, though it may improve the endurance of the fast-twitch fibers to a small degree.

Although aerobic capacity in leg muscles is vastly improved with training, the ability of the fibers to exercise with insufficient oxygen (anaerobic) may have changed little. The anaerobic capacity of both slow-twitch and fast-twitch fibers in distance runners is often below that found in untrained or strength-trained individuals. Several of the enzymes important in the anaerobic breakdown of glycogen are reduced or remain unchanged with endurance training. This may explain, in part, why distance runners find it difficult to sprint and produce little lactate when they attempt anaerobic running. In fact, distance runners' muscles seem better suited to using lactate for energy than they are at producing it.

These muscular adaptations make it clear that the gains during endurance training are specific to the speed and distance employed by the runner. While endurance training improves the aerobic capacity of the muscles, it reduces their ability to perform anaerobic or strength type activities. Strength training, on the other hand, produces no improvements in aerobic capacity, but it improves muscle power and anaerobic energy production. Football players and other anaerobically oriented athletes have remarkable strength and anaerobic tolerance, but they score no better than sedentary individuals in tests of aerobic capacity.

Despite the extensive reliance on the slow-twitch fibers during distance running, these fibers do not appear to grow any larger than the fast-twitch fibers during training. There is, however, considerable variability in the size of these muscle fibers among different runners. Some individuals have unusually large slow-twitch fibers, while other runners may have larger fast-twitch fibers. This point may be only of academic importance, since a runner's muscle size seems to have little relationship with performance. Muscle fiber size may be more critical in events that demand greater power and strength, such as sprint running and weightlifting.

Though most of our studies suggest that the percentage of slow-twitch and fast-twitch fibers does not change with distance running training, it now appears that during the initial stages of training muscle fiber characteristics may undergo some modifications. Modern techniques have enabled us to see some modifications in the contractile speed and power within the various fiber types. In Chapter 6 we will discuss the results of studies done with runners who have stopped running. In those cases, it appears that their fiber type shifts away from the high percentage of slow-twitch toward a more normal mixture of fast- and slow-twitch. In fact, it appears that many of the muscle fibers in sedentary and older people are a combination of slow-and fast-twitch fibers. These combination fibers are sometimes called hybrid fibers and can be detected using newer technologies with molecular biology that were not available 10 years ago. As a result, our understanding of muscle physiology and changes in fiber types with distance running is continuing to evolve.

Despite the variety of changes that occur in the leg muscles during training for distance running, the adaptations in elite runners differs little from those seen in less talented individuals. All individuals who train with the same volume and intensity will show some adaptations in muscle, regardless of their innate talents. This does not mean that less gifted individuals can achieve the performance level of those who were born with greater talents. Champions are born with the "right stuff" but must suffer the stresses of training to achieve their full potential. Those of us made of more mortal matter are limited to a greater degree by our genetic endowments that may control our ability to adapt to training.

DELIVERING OXYGEN

Shortness of breath, or the inability to ventilate the lungs, is perhaps the first signal of fatigue during exercise in untrained individuals. The muscles responsible for moving air in and out of the lungs are often as untrained as the leg muscles. Even during relatively slow running these muscles tire easily, making it difficult for the poorly conditioned runner to ventilate his/her lungs. Endurance training improves the endurance and strength of these muscles, enabling runners to easily move air in and out of the lungs, thereby unload carbon dioxide while replenishing oxygen to the blood. The sensation of shortness of breath is generally attributed to the build-up of carbon dioxide in the blood and respiratory centers of the brain. Consequently, when you are trained, rapid, deep breathing during distance running is easier, resulting in a greater ability to control the blood carbon dioxide levels.

Early studies showed few changes in the structure or function of the lung as a result of endurance training. Researchers observed only an increase in the rate of gas diffusion from the alveoli to the arterial blood as it passed through the lungs. Training increases the rate of blood flow through the lungs, delivering more blood in need of oxygen and removal of carbon dioxide. Thus, the oxygen gradient (difference) between the alveoli and the blood remains high, promoting a faster exchange of gases.

Upon leaving the lungs, arterial blood is nearly saturated (about 98%) with oxygen. Only during very intense, exhaustive running does the blood leave the lungs with less than a maximum load of oxygen. Since endurance training improves the ability of the respiratory muscles to move air in and out of the lungs, increases blood flow through the lungs, and enhances the rate at which oxygen can diffuse into the blood, runners are able to run faster and produce more energy without lowering the oxygen content of the blood.

The amount of oxygen carried by the blood is, in part, determined by the number of red blood cells and hemoglobin content of the blood. Several investigators have shown that a runner's $\dot{V}O_2$max is closely related to his or her red blood cell volume. Though training increases $\dot{V}O_2$max, there is little agreement regarding the effect of training on red cell volume or total hemoglobin content. Nevertheless, experts generally agree that years of training will increase the number of red blood cells without changing the amount of hemoglobin in each cell.

Physical activity also significantly increases the volume of plasma, the watery part of the blood. Though three weeks of bed rest will lower plasma volume by about 15%, one week of activity is sufficient to return it to normal. Endurance training will elevate plasma volume an additional 10 to 15%.

Without some increase in red cell volume, a rise in plasma volume will result in a marked dilution of the red cells. This may explain why some runners appear to be anemic at times during periods of hard training. They simply are experiencing a hemodilution caused by an expansion of their plasma. Nevertheless, some physiologists have suggested that red cells may be damaged or destroyed during intense physical exercise, lowering the oxygen-carrying capacity of the blood. Regardless of any fluctuations in red cell and plasma volumes, experts generally concede that total blood volume increases with training. Whether these changes are of significant magnitude to affect oxygen delivery to the muscles remains debatable.

BLOOD DOPING

Recently, some attention has been given to the use of blood reinfusion, sometimes termed "blood doping," to improve running performance. In theory, the addition of red blood cells to circulation might be expected to increase the oxygen-carrying capacity of blood, thereby improving a runner's $\dot{V}O_2$max. Swedish investigators, in the 1970s, observed that $\dot{V}O_2$max decreased by 13 to 18% when 400 to 800 ml of blood was withdrawn from well-trained men. Four weeks later, after their bodies had replaced the missing red cells, the blood was reinfused, thereby elevating the number of red cells and hemoglobin above normal. This procedure was found to improve physical performance capacity by 23% and $\dot{V}O_2$max by 9%. Although there have been some conflicting reports regarding the effects of blood reinfusion on endurance performance, physiologists generally agree that this procedure does increase oxygen transport and improve stamina. It should be pointed-out, however, that blood reinfusion exposes the athlete to several possible health risks, and is a procedure that has been banned by all athletic federations.

THE CARDIOVASCULAR SYSTEM AT WORK

In addition to improvements in the blood's capacity to carry oxygen, the major cardiovascular adaptation to training is an increased cardiac output, amount of blood pumped per minute, during maximal exercise. It is calculated by multiplying the heart rate by the stroke volume, which is the amount of blood ejected from the heart with each beat. Although cardiac output during less than maximal effort (submaximal) running is unaffected by training, there is a reduction in a runner's heart rate when he or she is running at a set pace. A slower exercising heart rate can only occur if the stroke volume (amount of blood pushed from the heart with each beat) increases. The following example illustrates how cardiac output can be the same during submaximal running both before and after training, with a lower heart rate.

$$\text{Cardiac Output} = (\text{stroke volume}) \times (\text{heart rate})$$

$$(\text{untrained}) \ 10,000 \ \text{ml/min} = (80 \ \text{ml/beat}) \times (125 \ \text{beats/min})$$

$$(\text{trained}) \ 10,000 \ \text{ml/min} = (100 \ \text{ml/beat}) \times (100 \ \text{beats/min})$$

The cause for this increase in the heart's stroke volume during both submaximal and maximal exercise is often attributed to an enlargement or hypertrophy of the heart with endurance training. The increase in heart size often seen in endurance athletes is the result of an enlarged ventricular cavity, but there is little increase in the thickening of the ventricular wall, the heart chambers that pump blood through the arteries. This means that the volume of blood that fills the ventricles and is pumped out of the heart is also larger. It should be noted, however, that heart volume does not always increase following physical training. Nevertheless, the ventricles may be stronger and able to empty their contents more fully as a consequence of endurance training. These changes in ventricular structure and function are responsible for the lower resting and submaximal heart rates observed among distance runners.

Maximal heart rate, on the other hand, may show little change with training. With the same maximal heart rate and an enlarged stroke volume, the total amount of blood pumped by the heart or maximal cardiac output during exhaustive exercise is greater in the trained runner.

It has been suggested that maximal stroke volume is the most distinguishing difference between champion endurance athletes and well-trained individuals. As mentioned, the increased stroke volume following training is, in part, achieved by an increase in blood volume. The late Steve Prefontaine, holder of numerous American distance running records, had a heart volume of 1,205 milliliters, approximately 30 to 40% larger than the average-sized heart of a man of equal age, height, and weight.

Training for distance running results in a combination of respiratory, circulatory, and muscular adaptations directed toward a greater capacity to produce energy and sustain muscular effort for long periods. The accumulated effect of all these physiological changes is an increase in $\dot{V}O_2$max. Though the magnitude of the increase in $\dot{V}O_2$max varies considerably, an improvement of 5 to 20% can be anticipated for individuals older than 16 years who initially train for eight to 12 weeks. As shown in Figure 4-3, the amount of improvement in $\dot{V}O_2$max is determined partly by the amount of training performed by the runner. In the example, the untrained runner has a $\dot{V}O_2$max of 40 milliliters of oxygen per minute for each kilogram of body weight (ml/kg × min). Training for several months at 25 miles per week results in a 12 ml/kg × min increase; when the training was doubled to 50 miles per week there was an additional rise of six to 7 ml/kg × min. The first reaction to such findings is to conclude that $\dot{V}O_2$max will continue to improve simply by increasing the training mileage. Unfortunately, the secrets of training are not so simple or straightforward.

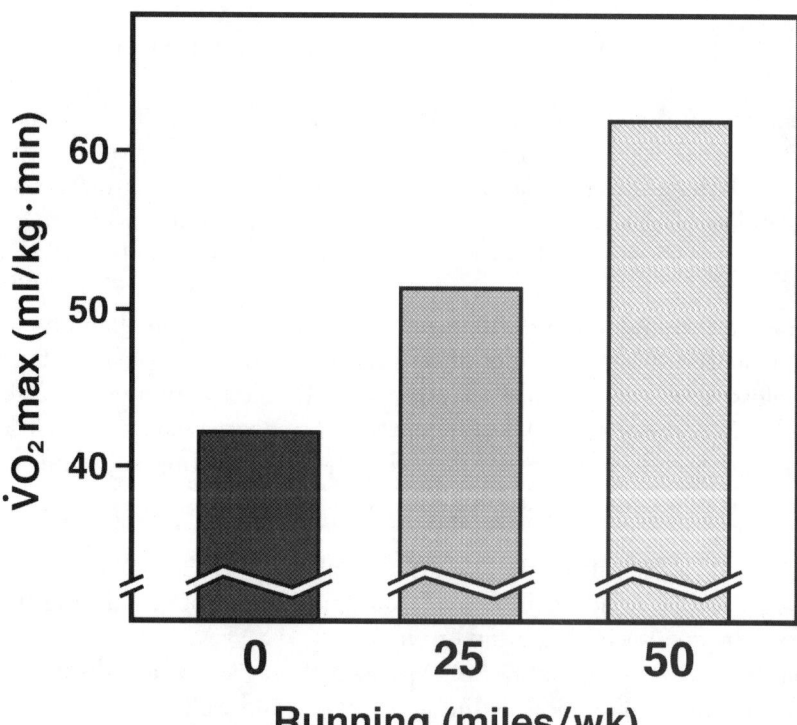

Figure 4-3. Maximal oxygen uptake for a 40-year-old man in the untrained state and after several months of training at 25 and 50 miles per week.

THE MILEAGE GAME

As noted in the previous figure, improvements in aerobic capacity are, in part, determined by the distance covered each week during training and the total mileage performed over several weeks. Many runners have learned to gauge their readiness for competition on the basis of their weekly mileage. Conversations among distance runners inevitably turn to "How many miles per week have you been running?" While most runners think that the more miles you run, the better your chances of success, it is easy to overtrain and perform poorly. **It is important to remember that the purpose of training is to stress the body, so that when you rest it will grow stronger and more tolerant of the demands of distance running.** Unfortunately, most runners forget that you can train too hard, or allow too little rest, which overstresses the body and minimizes opportunity for growth.

Some years ago at our laboratory we studied two marathon runners following a six-month layoff when they were at different stages in their reconditioning. Muscle biopsies and treadmill tests for $\dot{V}O_2$max were made as they gradually increased their weekly mileage. As one might have predicted, the muscles showed dramatic improvements in aerobic capacity with as little as 25 miles of running per week. Figure 4-4 shows that the runners' $\dot{V}O_2$max values increased when they progressively increased their training to 75 miles per week. Beyond that level of training, however, our laboratory tests found no additional gains in

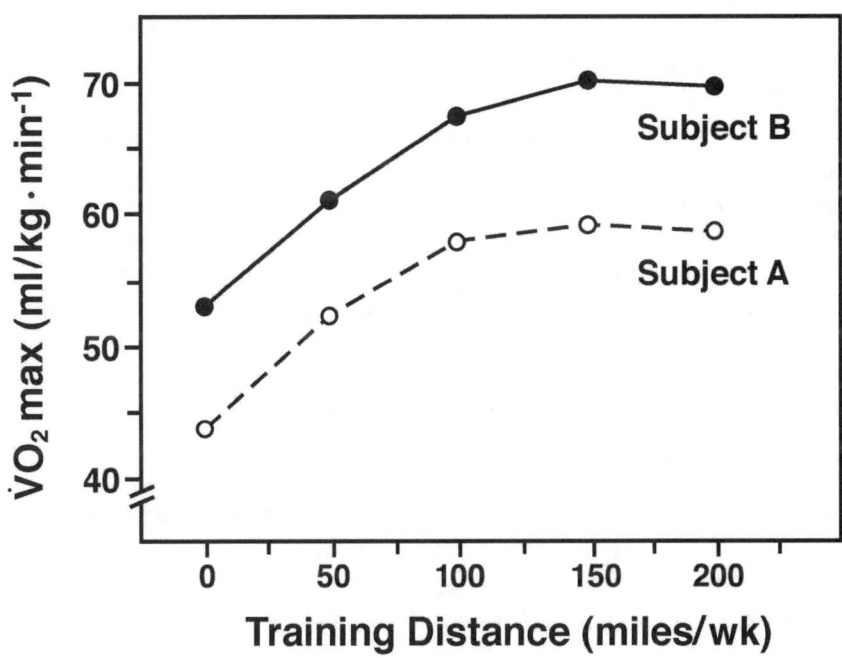

Figure 4-4. *Changes in $\dot{V}O_2$max for two distance runners while training at various distances. Note that training 50 to 100 miles per week resulted in significant improvements in $\dot{V}O_2$max, whereas greater training distances produced no greater increases.*

endurance. During a one-month period they even trained at 225 miles per week, with no improvement in endurance.

The efforts of such crazy students and other studies with swimmers, who also tend to train in excess, have led us to realize that it is possible to overload the body's system for training adaptation. There is a point of optimal distance that will cause the body to adapt to its full aerobic capacity. Unfortunately, that optimal mileage is probably different for everyone. George Sheehan once said, "If five guys are training together, there is probably only one of them that might be training at the optimal distance and pace." Though we cannot write a cookbook for training that will suit everyone, it is reasonable to assume that, on average, maximum training benefits can be achieve with mileage of 60 to 90 miles per week. There is a point of diminishing return, a point at which you can increase weekly mileage but see little or no improvement in performance.

If you are currently training at 25 to 40 miles per week, there may be physiological advantages to be gained from additional mileage, but there are also pitfalls to avoid. **Don't increase your mileage too fast!** The body can tolerate slightly greater amounts of stress, but too much too fast will lead to a breakdown in adaptation rather than gains. Most runners can tolerate a 5 to 10% increase in their weekly mileage without becoming chronically fatigued. If, for example, you are already doing 50 miles per week, you may be able to increase the mileage by three to five miles without overdoing it.

In light of the previous discussion regarding the use and replacement of muscle and liver glycogen, the training regimen should allow for adequate recovery. Most runners attempt to train hard every day, with the idea that the more they do, the better they will be. Running the same distance at the same pace each day does not allow the runner's body to recover sufficiently and offers little opportunity to inject any quality or speed into the training program.

The rate at which the body adapts to the training stimulus is relatively slow, because many of the adaptations require the restructuring of various protein components of the muscles. The benefits gained from a given workout may not be realized for several weeks, since protein turnover is a slow process. No, it doesn't speed things up to eat more protein! The training regimen should be planned over a three- or four-week period, rather than day-to-day or week-by-week. Be gradual in your training progression.

Although you have to stress the body hard to raise your exercise tolerance to a new and better level of fitness, once you have gained the benefits of increased mileage, you can reduce your training without losing anything. In fact, after training for a few weeks at 60-plus miles you can probably perform better by decreasing your total weekly mileage to 40 or 50 miles. Our studies have shown that you can perform at your best only during two- to six-week periods of reduced training. During that period, however, you still need to have one long training run every week or two. Whereas this might mean a 20-mile run for the marathoner, a 10-mile run should satisfy the specific needs of a 10-kilometer runner. These long runs appear to develop and maintain the muscles' aerobic energy systems, specifically the abilities to use fat and spare the use of muscle glycogen.

How do runners train? A survey of today's runners reveals that 60% run 45 to 52 miles per week, while nearly 40% run more than 100 miles per week. On the average, elite U.S. distance runners train at 100 to 150 miles per week. This contrasts with some elite runners of earlier periods. Alfred Shrubb, who in 1904 ran 50min:50s for the 10-mile, and 9min:09.8s for the two-mile, covered only 35 miles of moderate running per week. Walter George, world record holder for the mile (4 min:10.8s) in 1882, reported that he ran fewer than 10 miles per week, most of it at a relatively slow pace. Training was more intense for the runners at the 1962 Western Hemisphere Marathon, where those who finished among the leaders trained year-round, twice per day, and ran more than 100 miles per week.

What are your goals? If running for fitness is your goal, then 20 to 25 miles per week may be plenty. Those who want to compete in 5 and 10K races might do better on 35 to 40 miles per week. Whereas, those crazy enough to torture themselves during a marathon would best prepare with mileage of 60 to 90 miles per week. Both experience and scientific evidence suggests that optimal training distance for maximal endurance development demands between 60 to 90 miles per week. Runners who are less tolerant of heavy training may achieve greater benefits from training at less than 60 miles per week, where they minimize the risk of overstress.

PACE: THE SPEED OF TRAINING

Although the volume of running during training, rather than the speed, is the most important determinant for developing aerobic endurance, distance racing success also depends to a large degree on the quality, or speed, of training. The major disadvantage of concentrating on "volume" in a training program is that long, slow distance training is considerably slower than racing pace. Such training fails to develop the neurological patterns of muscle fiber recruitment that will be needed during races that require a faster pace. Since the selective use of muscle fibers differs according to running speed, runners who only train at speeds slower than race pace will not train all of the muscle fibers or efficiency needed for competition. We have found that these individuals show marked improvements in performance when they race frequently. This suggests that the faster speeds of competition supplement the runners' aerobic endurance with patterns of movement that make their running more efficient.

INTERVAL TRAINING: AEROBIC

How can you train at a faster pace, and still put in the mileage? High-intensity training may include either intermittent running, known as intervals, or continuous running at a somewhat faster pace. Although interval training has been used for many years, most runners who use interval training try to run at too fast a pace, with long rest intervals. While some interval training can be performed at speeds that produce large lactate accumulations, it is also possible to use this training format to enhance the aerobic system. Repeated runs at slightly faster pace, over shorter distances, with brief rest intervals will achieve the same benefits as long continuous runs. This form of "**aerobic interval**" training has become the framework for aerobic swimming conditioning. It involves repeated short swims at slightly slower than race pace with very brief rest intervals of five to 15 seconds.

Table 4.2 offers an example of some **aerobic intervals** for runners who are preparing to compete in a 10-kilometer race. Since volume is the key to successful aerobic training, the runner must perform a large number of these repeated runs. In this example, 20 repetitions of 400 meters results in a total of 8,000 meters or roughly five miles. The pace is five to six seconds per minute slower than that maintained during a 10-kilometer race, but it is generally faster than a speed that could be sustained easily during a straight five-mile run. The hard part of this interval set is that the prescribed rest between repetitions is relatively brief, 10 to 30 seconds. These short rest intervals keep the circulatory system working at a relatively high level, yet give the runner a brief escape from the muscular stress of the faster running.

Figure 4-5 illustrates a runner's heart rate and oxygen uptake while running a set of five 800-meter aerobic intervals. There is little recovery of either heart rate or oxygen uptake during the 15-second rest intervals, with energy levels at 73% of the runner's $\dot{V}O_2$max. Little or no lactate accumulated in the blood of this runner, suggesting that she was able to perform the interval set without demanding energy from the anaerobic metabolism. One advantage of this form of

TABLE 4-2. Example of aerobic intervals for runners training to run a 10-kilometer race.

Best 10-km min:sec	Interval Set			
	Reps	Distance (meters)	Rest (sec)	Pace (min:sec)
46:00	20	400	10–15	2:00
43:00	20	400	10–15	1:52
40:00	20	400	10–15	1:45
37:00	20	400	10–15	1:37
34:00	20	400	10–15	1:30

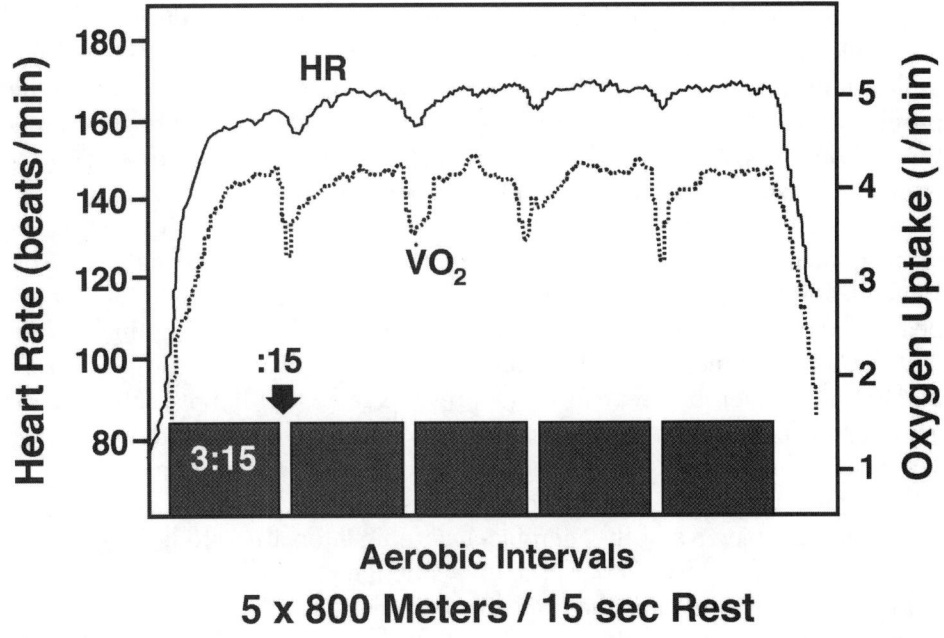

Figure 4-5. *Heart rate and oxygen uptake (V̇O₂) during a series of aerobic interval runs with 15-second rests between each run.*

training is that the runner can systematically increase the training load and plot his or her improvement.

It can be argued that a straight run of five miles at a similar pace will give the same aerobic benefits, but some runners find this form of training lacking in stimulation. When it comes to the aerobic aspects of training, personal preference can be the deciding factor. Whether you prefer one hard run of five or 6 miles or a series of repeated, short runs with brief rest intervals, the aerobic benefits will be the same.

INTERVAL TRAINING: RACE PACE

To train the leg muscles to produce the force required for racing and to co-ordinate the various muscles involved in running fast, a portion of the runner's training should be performed at or near racing pace. By far the most effective way to accomplish this goal is to perform interval sets at speeds approximating race pace, referred to as "**aerobic-anaerobic intervals**." These near-race pace intervals have also been termed "aerobic threshold intervals". Generally, these intervals cause little or no accumulation of blood lactate when running at marathon pace intervals. Preparing for races like the mile, 5K, or even 10K may produce some accumulation of blood lactate, but generally this does not become a limiting factor.

Shown in Figure 4-6 are heart rate and oxygen uptake values during aerobic-anaerobic interval sets run at marathon pace and at 10K pace. The lactate accumulation in the blood during these intervals is shown in Figure 4-7. Unlike the purely "aerobic intervals," these repeated race-pace runs require greater energy production rates of between 80 and 95% $\dot{V}O_2max$, resulting in some lactate accumulation and heart rates above 160 beats per minute.

Although we must emphasize that it is very misleading and often inaccurate to suggest a pace chart for interval training, we thought Table 4-3 might give you some idea of the speeds one "might" hope to run during a set of 400-meter repeats. The paces shown are based on the runners' best 10-kilometer times. Note that the total distance covered (4,000 meters) is less than that covered during the 400-meter "aerobic" repeats in the previous table, but the rest intervals are greater to allow for recovery from these faster runs. Though the rest intervals shown in the 400-meter interval sets are 60 to 90 seconds, experience and conditioning will help runners judge how much rest is needed.

Since the objective of the "aerobic-anaerobic intervals" is to develop speed and to learn the feel for proper pace, only enough rest to enable the runner to hold the desired pace for all the runs should be allowed. If fatigue during the latter runs forces a reduction in pace, then either the rest interval is too brief or the pace is too fast. The pre-selected pace for these interval runs should not be faster than what is realistic for the runner's anticipated pace during the race. The key to success in aerobic-anaerobic interval training is to manipulate the rest interval, so that eventually the repeated runs are performed at racing speed with rests of only 30 to 45 seconds.

This form of interval training will also produce maximal gains in aerobic endurance, but it is too stressful to perform more than twice or three times per week. Since this form of training produces some lactate accumulation and a rapid breakdown of muscle glycogen, day-to-day recovery will be slower than during continuous and aerobic interval training. When a coach or a runner design sets of aerobic-anaerobic intervals, the running pace should be constant at racing speed, regardless of the distance covered during each run.

TABLE 4-3. Example of aerobic-anaerobic intervals for runners training to run a 10-kilometer race.

Best 10-km min:sec	Interval Set			
	Reps	Distance (meters)	Rest (sec)	Pace (min:sec)
46:00	10	400	60–90	1:51
43:00	10	400	60–90	1:44
40:00	10	400	60–90	1:37
37:00	10	400	60–90	1:29
34:00	10	400	60–90	1:16

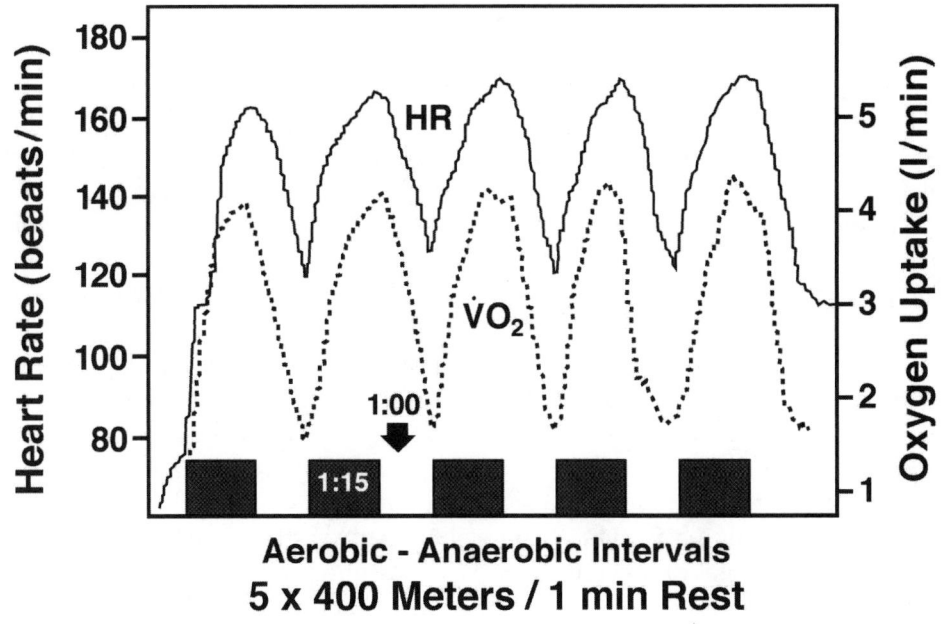

Figure 4-6. *Oxygen uptake and heart rate during aerobic-anaerobic intervals run at marathon and 10-kilometer paces. This runner's best performance for these events were 3h:21 min and 40 min:18s, respectively.*

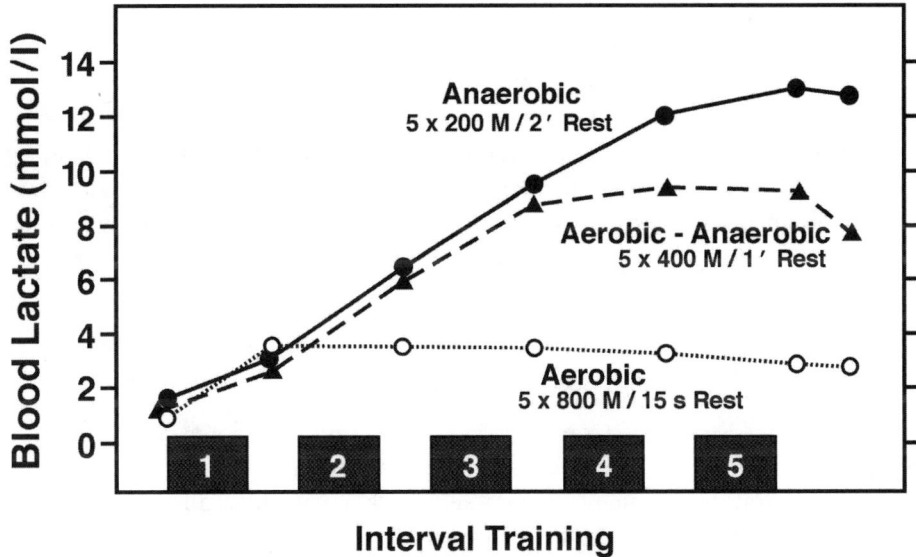

Figure 4-7. *Blood lactate accumulation during aerobic, aerobic-anaerobic, and anaerobic interval training. Note that despite the very short rest intervals of 15 seconds provided during the aerobic intervals, very little lactate accumulated. The longer rest intervals of two minutes and faster running speeds of the anaerobic intervals, on the other hand, resulted in a large lactate accumulation.*

ANAEROBIC INTERVAL TRAINING

Speed training is by far the most stressful form of muscular exercise. The energy for sprint running is derived, in large part, from the anaerobic break-down of muscle glycogen, which places great stress on the muscle's contractile filaments, fiber membranes and connective tissue (i.e., fascia and tendons). While these stresses improve strength and speed, there is also a greater risk of muscle injury due to the high tension generated during each run. Warming-up and mild stretching before these interval runs are a must. It is also wise to per-form the first of the runs a bit slower than the average time for the set.

The primary objective of these anaerobic intervals is to improve the runner's leg strength and to develop the ability to remove lactate from the muscles, thereby enhancing the runner's tolerance for faster than race-pace running. In light of the stress on the muscles during anaerobic interval training, there should be fewer repetitions and longer rests than there are in other forms of interval training. This training is aimed at developing strength and not aerobic en-durance, so the total distance covered is not as important. Since much of the energy produced during these interval runs will be produced anaerobically, there is a build-up of acid within the muscle, leading to early exhaustion if the pace is too fast and/or the rest intervals are too short.

Figure 4-8 shows some of the data from a runner we monitored while per-forming a set of ten 200-meter anaerobic intervals. Despite rests of two minutes between the runs, blood lactate, heart rate, and oxygen uptake were nearly at maximum during the final repetitions.

Although the example shown in Table 4-4 may help to gauge the proper pace for a set of anaerobic intervals, the final decision on a running pace be-comes a matter of experience and conditioning. Like other forms of strength training, this muscle overloading should not be repeated on successive days, and no more than one or two such training sessions should be performed in any seven-day training plan.

TRAINING PLAN

Though we have discussed some of the building blocks of a training pro-gram, it is probably not clear how these forms of training fit together to promote optimal preparation for racing. How many days per week and how many times per day should one train? Most attempts to evaluate the impact of training fre-quency on endurance capacity has been limited to studies using previously sedentary subjects, which probably isn't a good basis for detailing a training pro-gram for an already fit runner. Nevertheless, studies have shown significant im-provements in $\dot{V}O_2$max with two or 4 exercise bouts per week, but after seven weeks, there were no differences between the two- and four-day per week train-

90   *RUNNING: THE ATHLETE WITHIN*

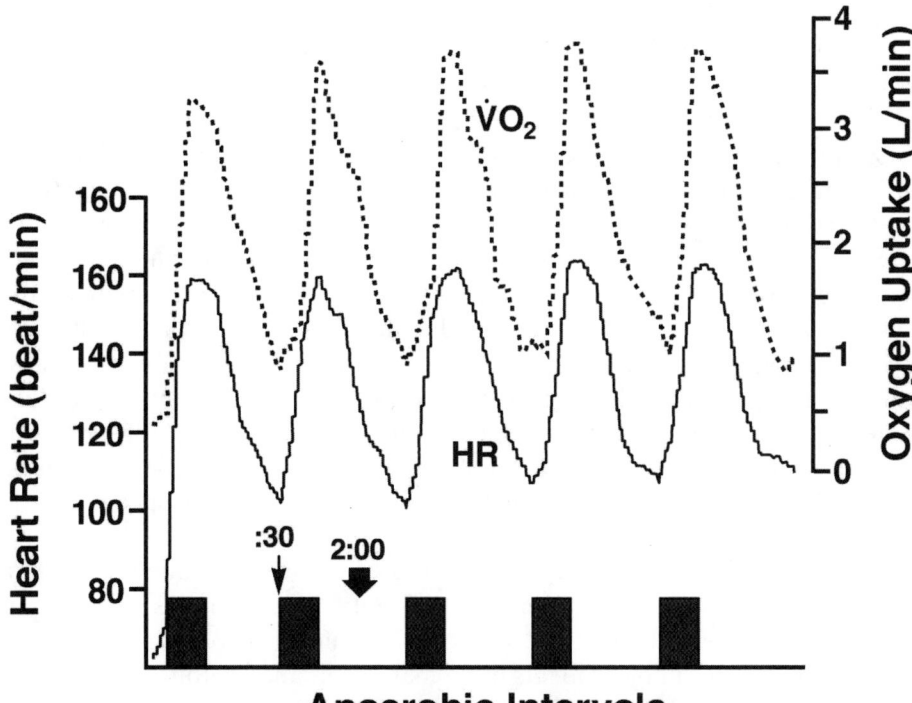

Figure 4-8. *Oxygen uptake and heart rate during a set of anaerobic sprint intervals.*

ing groups. After 20 weeks of training, however, the subjects who trained four days per week showed significantly greater gains in $\dot{V}O_2$max.

It is difficult to apply these data to already fit runners, whose training frequency and volume are substantially greater than those of the subjects used in the experimental studies. Judging from current training methods, the greatest gains in aerobic capacity are achieved when runners train four to 5 days per week.

The factors which determine the number of training sessions per week are: (1) the runner's state of training, (2) individual tolerance to training, and (3) the pace and distance of each training session. Even among highly trained runners, there are some who may respond better to training four days per week, while others may thrive on six or seven days per week with two daily training sessions. Individual differences in training tolerance are determined by each runner's recovery rate, that is the amount of rest needed between training sessions to allow for improvement.

During the early stages of conditioning, in periods following months or years of relative inactivity, the body is ill-prepared to meet the demands of hard exercise. The oxygen transport system is weak, muscle fuel supplies are low, and the ability to produce energy is poor. Consequently, it takes little exercise to stimulate new growth and improve endurance.

Unfortunately, most athletes believe that if they train hard and long, they will get into condition faster than they will with a less stressful program. Body tissues have an optimal rate of adaptation to training. When the training stress is either too small or too great, the rate of adaptation is lower and the conditioning is slower than desired. So, it is not wise to attempt a training program that is too demanding for your state of readiness of exercise. In other words, training twice per day will not get you into racing shape "twice as fast" as once per day!

Since it is impossible to prescribe the "optimal" training regimen for every beginning runner, it is prudent to design a training program that is more on the conservative side, and easily tolerated by the runner. The aim of this initial phase of conditioning is to stimulate a progressive increase in $\dot{V}o_2$max. Table 4-4 illustrates a training plan for the first four weeks of training, beginning in the "untrained" state. Though this regimen illustrates the need for a progressive increase in volume, the running pace is of less importance. As a rule, all of these sessions should be performed at conversational paces, which are speeds that do not cause the runner to feel short of breath.

This gradual progression in training distance should continue for the first eight weeks, reaching a maximum of 4 to 6 miles of continuous running per training session. Regardless of the frequency of training (two, four, or five days per week), the major improvements in $\dot{V}o_2$max are attained within the first eight weeks of training. This period is essential in establishing an "aerobic base" to prepare the runner for more intense training efforts.

10K TRAINING

The second stage of training, the preparation for competition, emphasizes the quality or pace of training, with small increments in training distance. At this point, both the training distance and speed of running are determined by the runner's planned racing distance. If the runner is preparing for a marathon, the

TABLE 4-4. A four-week training plan for the beginning runner, after a long period of inactivity. The "m" denotes miles covered in each training session, and the "°" indicates that each run may be performed as intermittent running and walking to keep the session exclusively aerobic.

	Days of Training						
	Day 1	Day 2	Day 3	Day 4	Day 5	Day 6	Day 7
Week 1	1 m°	1 m°	Rest	1.5 m°	1.5 m°	Rest	Rest
Week 2	1.5 m°	1 m	Rest	1.5 m	1.5 m	Rest	Rest
Week 3	2 m	1.5 m	Rest	2 m	1.5 m	Rest	2 m
Week 4	2 m	Rest	2.5 m	2 m	Rest	2.5 m	2 m

total daily mileage should gradually be increased to 8 or 10 miles with one extra long, aerobic run of 15 to 20 miles every week or two. Training for 10,000 meters, on the other hand, requires more of the aerobic-anaerobic type of training, with a maximum training distance of six or eight miles per session. The longest weekly run should not exceed 10 to 12 miles, at a strictly aerobic pace.

Table 4-5 illustrates an eight-week training plan, showing the mixture of aerobic, aerobic-anaerobic, and anaerobic training for 10-kilometer racing. To improve both aerobic capacity and leg power, the weekly training sessions provide a gradual increase in mileage and training pace. Since the aerobic-anaerobic and anaerobic training sessions tend to impose more stress on the energy reserves, allowances must be made for aerobic training on days following these sessions. This progression also allows for weekly variations in stress. This training plan recommends a three-week cycle, with progressive increments in mileage. Note that the longest mileage weeks of training are followed by a week of reduced effort.

In addition to the interval training sessions shown in the Table 4-5, each workout should start with one to 2 miles of easy, aerobic running. Although the scientific documentation on the value of warm-up is unclear, a slow entry into

TABLE 4-5. A sample training plan for 10-kilometer competition. Abbreviations Ae (aerobic), Ae-An (aerobic-anaerobic), and An (anaerobic) denote the training emphasis for that day. Refer to Tables 4-1, 4-2, and 4-3 for an explanation of the pace and rest used with the sample interval set shown below the Ae-An and An sessions.

	Day 1	Day 2	Day 3	Day 4	Day 5	Day 6	Day 7
Week 1	Ae 6 m	Ae-An 10 × 800	Ae 6 m	Rest	Ae-An 20 × 400	Ae 6 m	Rest
Week 2	Ae 8 m	Ae-An 5 × 1,500	Ae 6 m	Rest	Ae 7 m	Ae-An 6 × 1,200	Rest
Week 3	Ae 9 m	Ae-An 15 × 600	Rest	An 10 × 200	Ae 7 m	Ae-An 6 × 800	Rest
Week 4	Ae 6 m	Ae-An 10 × 400	Rest	Ae 6 m	Ae-An 3 × 1,500	Ae 5 m	Rest
Week 5	Ae 8 m	Ae-An 5 × 1,200	Ae 6 m	An 5 × 400	Ae-An 15 × 600	Ae 7 m	Rest
Week 6	Ae 10 m	Ae-An 40 × 200	Ae 7 m	An 7 × 300	Ae-An 6 × 1,000	Ae 7 m	Rest
Week 7	Ae 8 m	Ae-An 8 × 800	Ae 6 m	Rest 6 m	Ae 4 × 1,500	Ae-An	Rest
Week 8	Ae 10 m	An 6 × 400	Ae-An 2 × 4,000	Ae 6 m	An 10 × 200	Ae-An 5 × 1,200	Rest

"m" denotes miles, whereas the interval sets are described as the number of repetitions and the distance in meters (10 reps × 400 meters).

the intense portion of the workout will lessen the risk of injury and permit some physiological adjustment to the energy demands of hard exercise.

The value of warming-down is debatable. Many coaches and runners recommend one to two miles of easy running at the end of the training session. Recovery from a highly anaerobic training bout will be faster if the runner continues to do some easy aerobic running. The rate of lactate removal from the blood is faster with an "active recovery" than it is when the subject stops exercise. There is, however, evidence that some of the muscle glycogen used during intense exercise is replaced from lactate after the exercise. You can see in Figure 4-9 that continued muscular activity after an intense sprint bout produces an additional breakdown of muscle glycogen, whereas complete inactivity results in 50 to 75% recovery. This would lead us to conclude that during repeated days of intense training, it may be better to avoid warming-down, in order to reduce the day-to-day loss of muscle glycogen. Before we get too radical, it might be wise to stay with tradition. A little easy exercise might speed recovery from the fatigue, though that point is still debatable.

MARATHON TRAINING

Several major adjustments must be made in the preceding training plan to accommodate the specific adaptations needed for marathon running. There are, however, more similarities than differences in the 10-kilometer and marathon training programs. This may explain why many of the best marathoners have years of training and competitive experience as 10-kilometer runners. The

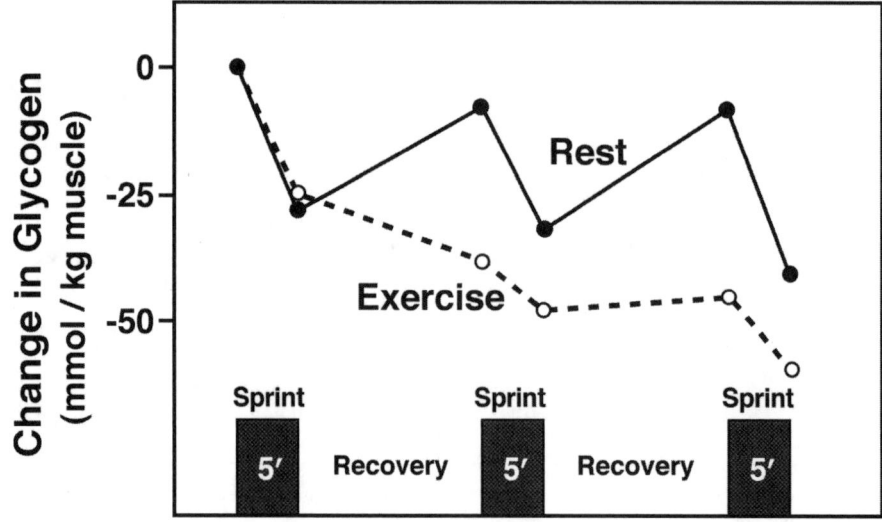

Figure 4-9. *Effect of active (exercise) and inactive (rest) recovery following five minutes of sprint exercise. Note that muscle glycogen decreases with each sprint bout, then continues to decline when the runners perform light activity during the recovery. Complete rest after the sprint bouts, on the other hand, results in a marked recovery of muscle glycogen.*

marathon requires more emphasis on aerobic endurance than on leg speed and power, but it is still a race against time. Consequently, the difference between surviving the distance and performing one's best will be determined by the runner's efficiency and specific leg strength. As we have pointed out in the preceding chapters, specificity is a key consideration in all forms of training. Training only at speeds slower than one's racing pace will not fully prepare the energy, circulatory, and neurological systems for the demands of competition.

Some definite compromises must be made to accommodate the special demands of the marathon. If we compare the proposed training regimen for the 10K and that of the marathon (Table 4-6), it is evident that the amount of intense (aerobic-anaerobic) training remains relatively constant from week to week, but the total volume and longest weekly training runs increase within each three-week cycle. The aerobic interval sets shown in this table are performed with short rest intervals and at speeds slower than racing pace. The aerobic-anaerobic intervals, on the other hand, are run at the desired racing pace, but with substantially longer rest intervals. Again, the aerobic-anaerobic intervals should be preceded by a one- to two-mile easy warm-up run. This plan is designed to provide progressive, yet specific training for the marathon. Remember that the physiological adaptations to training are relatively slow, it seems that this phase of training will require eight to 12 weeks for optimal benefits.

The training plan presented in Table 4-6 is an example and should be modified to suit individual abilities, racing distances, and responses to each form of

TABLE 4-6. A sample training plan for marathon competition. Abbreviations Ae (aerobic) and Ae-An (aerobic-anaerobic) denote the training emphasis for each day. Refer to Tables 4-1 and 4-2 for an explanation of the pace and rest used with the sample interval sets shown below in the Ae-An sessions.

	Day 1	Day 2	Day 3	Day 4	Day 5	Day 6	Day 7
Week 1	Ae 8 m	Ae 6×1 m	Ae-An 10×800	Ae 4 m	Ae 8 m	Ae-An 20×400	Rest
Week 2	Ae 10 m	Ae 3×2 m	Ae-An 15×600	Ae 5 m	Ae-An 8×1 m	Ae 8 m	Rest
Week 3	Ae 12 m	Ae-An 8×1 m	Ae 2×4 m	Ae 6 m	Ae-An 20×400	Ae 9 m	Rest
Week 4	Ae 9 m	Ae 6×1.5m	Ae-An 10×800	Ae 5 m	Ae 9 m	Ae-An 15×600	Rest
Week 5	Ae 11 m	Ae 4×2 m	Ae-An 8×1 m	Ae 6 m	Ae-An 20×400	Ae 9 m	Rest
Week 6	Ae 14 m	Ae-An 30×300	Ae 2×5 m	Ae 7 m	Ae-An $9 \times 1,000$	Ae 10 m	Rest

"m" denotes miles, whereas the interval sets are described as the number of repetitions and distance in meters (10 reps × 400 meters).

training. The distance and number of repetitions illustrated in the various forms of interval training can be increased or decreased to provide variety and to modify the volume of training. Although the examples provide some basis for 10-kilometer and marathon running, the same plans can be modified to help the runner prepare for most racing distances. The traditional approach to training distance runners generally focused only on the importance of increasing the runner's weekly mileage. There is now sound evidence to show that the quality of training is equally as important as the quantity.

STRENGTH TRAINING FOR DISTANCE RUNNING

Although distance running improves muscular endurance, there is some research evidence that it may produce a decline in leg strength. As noted in Chapter 1, distance runners lack the ability to sprint and jump. Recent studies with single muscle fiber taken from biopsies of distance runners have shown that their fibers are smaller and less powerful than non-runners. These findings are in keeping with the knowledge that endurance training reduces the maximal tension in muscle. Since running speed depends on specific leg strength, such decrements in muscle power tend to negate the full benefit of training for peak performance. As a result, many runners have incorporated some form of strength training into their training programs in an attempt to compensate for their apparent loss in explosive leg strength and speed.

Although there are numerous anecdotal reports describing the benefits of strength training for distance running, there is no scientific evidence to support this practice. Those runners who engage in strength training most frequently use free weights, hand-held weights, ankle weights, and weighted vests. These methods differ only in the way that they impose additional overloads to the muscle.

Free weights, for example, tend to isolate specific leg and arm actions in an effort to strengthen the muscles used during distance running. The major fault with this approach is that any strength gained while working against a given piece of strength equipment is not transferred to the task of running. The runner may be able to lift a heavier weight or exert greater force, but there is no assurance that he or she will be able to run faster or easier. The problem is specificity. Unless the strength training is done while the runner is running, it is not likely to be beneficial.

Based on this principle, some runners elect to add resistance to the muscles by wearing weights to the trunk, arms, or legs. The addition of a pound of weight to the ankle, for example, is equivalent to adding four pounds to the trunk. In theory, these methods would seem to offer a more specific approach to improve strength and speed, but the benefits are undocumented. The major disadvantage of these methods is that adding weights to the body tends to change one's running style and increase the chance for injury and joint stress. Because it costs a runner more to carry the added weight, he or she will be forced to run slower while working at the same relative effort (%$\dot{V}O_2$max). Being forced to run slower by the addition of weights works in opposition to the principle of specificity: to race fast you must, within reason, train fast. Strength gained during slow running will not insure strength gains for racing. Running with weights provides no greater training stimulus for the oxygen transport system than running without the use of added weight. If you want to train at a higher percentage of your $\dot{V}O_2$max, then you need to run faster. We are not saying, however, that every training session should be performed at sprint speed! No, we'd prefer that the training sessions be controlled, as described previously.

Thus, the most specific method for strength training is to overload the muscles while running at increased speeds for short distances. The strength needed for long distance running is not the same as that demanded by power events like weightlifting. Nevertheless, the training principles are much the same. The load on the muscles must be near maximum for very brief periods. Anaerobic interval training is designed to promote strength gains that are directly transferable to improvements in leg speed. Since leg speed and strength are of diminishing importance during races of greater and greater distance, the emphasis on anaerobic intervals should be virtually eliminated from training regimens for races greater than 10 to 12 miles. Since this form of training is highly taxing, it should be used no more than three days per week. Even within a given training session, the amount of anaerobic (sprint) training should make up only about 10% of the total daily mileage.

WARM WEATHER TRAINING

No single factor threatens the health and performance of the distance runner as much as a hot, sunny, humid day. The ability to compete well in hot weather depends, in part, on prior training in the heat. Prolonged and repeated training runs in the heat gradually improve your ability to eliminate excess body heat, reducing the risk of heat exhaustion and heat stroke. This process, termed "heat acclimation," results in a number of adjustments in the distribution of blood flow and sweating. Though the amount of sweat produced during exercise in the heat does not always change with heat acclimatization, the distribution of sweating over the skin often increases in those areas that have the greatest exposure and are most effective in dissipating body heat.

Heat acclimatization is generally characterized by reductions in heart rate and rectal temperature during exercise in the heat. These physiological adjustments improve rapidly with successive days of training in the heat, being fully improved within eight to 12 days. Heat acclimatization depends on the running speed, the duration of heat exposure, and the environmental conditions during each exercise session.

Laboratory studies have frequently required runners to exercise at a low intensity of about 50% $\dot{V}O_2$max for 80 to 100 minutes in a chamber heated to between 90 and 120°F to induce a full heat adjustment. Unfortunately, there is no information to show the rate and degree of acclimatization during short training runs of 30 to 60 minutes at higher intensities of 70 to 80% $\dot{V}O_2$max. Nevertheless, the physiological responses of trained runners suggest that they are quite tolerant of hot weather running, as long as at least part of their training is performed in the heat. As with all other forms of training, the adjustments to the heat are specific to the conditions. Heat acclimatization can only be achieved by exercising in the heat, not by enjoying passive activities such as sunbathing.

Figure 4-10 illustrates the adjustments in a runner's heart rate and rectal temperature during 90 minutes of exercise at 60% $\dot{V}O_2$max in heat of 102°F before and after eight days of heat acclimatization. Although some investigators have reported decreases in oxygen uptake during exercise in the heat, we have observed only minor changes in the rate of energy and heat production as a consequence of acclimatization.

Improved heat tolerance is associated with an earlier onset of sweating at the beginning of exercise. As a result, skin temperature is lower, and the difference between the temperatures of body and skin is greater. Thus, less blood flow

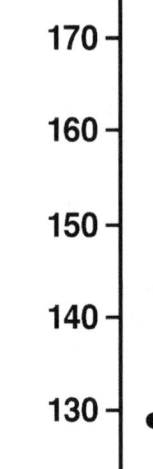

Figure 4-10. Heart rate and rectal temperature during 90 minutes of exercise in the heat (102 degrees Fahrenheit) before and after eight days of heat acclimatization. Note the lower recording after training in the heat.

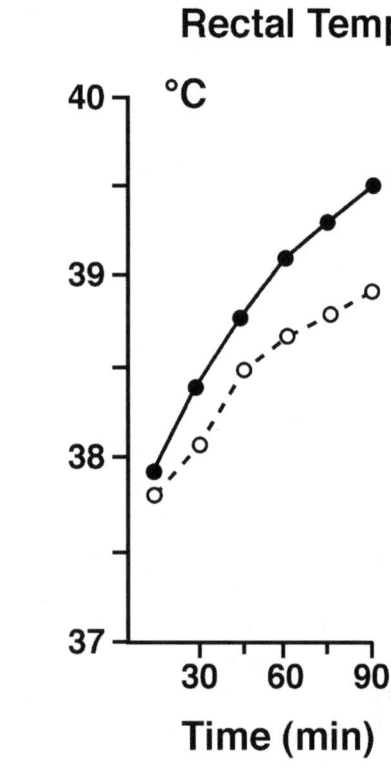

to the skin is required to transfer excess body heat. Although some investigators have found an increase in blood volume with heat acclimatization, this change is somewhat temporary. It is probably related to the body's efforts to retain sodium, which causes the body to retain more water.

What does all this mean to distance runners, and how can they train to gain the greatest degree of heat acclimatization? Although runners must be exposed to the heat to fully adjust, they gain partial heat tolerance by training in a cooler environment. In addition, when the runners become acclimatized to a given level of heat stress, they will also be able to perform better in cooler weather. If the runner must compete in hot weather, then at least part of the training should be conducted in the warmest part of the day. Early morning and evening training runs will not fully prepare a distance runner to tolerate the heat of midday.

One possible side effect of running in the heat is the stress it places on muscle glycogen stores. Running at a given speed in the heat will require a greater use of muscle glycogen than the same run in cooler air. As a result, repeated days of training in the heat may cause a rapid depletion of muscle glycogen and the symptoms of chronic fatigue. Heat acclimatization reduces this rate of glycogen use by as much as 50 to 60%, thereby reducing the risk of exhaustion due to a depletion of the muscle's energy reserves.

Runners must guard against injuries such as heat stroke and heat exhaustion. Heat acclimatization cannot be accelerated by avoiding water during training. You cannot adapt to dehydration! Taking fluids will minimize the hazards of heat injury and enable you to train better.

TRAINING IN THE COLD

Some runners believe that the heat produced by exercise provides the necessary warmth for cold weather running. Since most runners lack the fatty insulation needed to retain body heat, this may not be the case. We have, on a number of occasions, observed rectal temperatures below resting levels in distance runners after long runs of 10 to 25 miles in temperatures ranging from 20 to 30°F. Although the runners were warmly clothed, rectal temperatures decreased from resting values of 99.2°F to less than 98°F.

Numerous investigators have found no evidence of cold acclimatization in humans. Some cold adjustment has been observed among men and women during resting conditions, but evidence is lacking concerning running performance and cold exposure.

While there is limited research to describe the effects of cold weather running on the distance runner, one might theorize that under extremely cold conditions, the quantity of heat loss may exceed that produced by the muscles. The risk of becoming hypothermic is greatest in long races where fatigue may force the runners to decrease their pace, which lowers the rate of body heat production. Although the distance runner tends to perform better under cool conditions, extreme body heat loss can cause the runner to weaken and even collapse.

Despite low environmental temperatures, men have been found to sweat profusely, which causes substantial weight loss and surprisingly low skin temperature. Accumulation of sweat in the clothing and on the skin provides a rapid mechanism for heat loss by conduction to the cold, wet microenvironment surrounding the runner.

Other major threats posed by running in subfreezing air are those associated with frostbite and irritations to the respiratory tract. The wind chill imposed by running increases the risk of freezing injuries. Though such injuries to the skin may occur at temperatures barely below freezing, irritations and tissue damage to the respiratory tract seldom occur when the temperature is above 10°F. Experts generally agree that training and racing should not be attempted below 10 to 1°F.

TRAINING FOR ALTITUDE

Much of the preceding discussion has described the human capacity to perform endurance exercise under relatively compatible climatic conditions. However, the atmosphere that provides the oxygen needed for aerobic energy production is not uniform. Running is markedly influenced by the reduced oxygen content of the air at high altitudes.

The exchange of oxygen between the air sacs of the lungs and the blood passing through the lungs depends on the difference in the number of oxygen molecules available in the lungs and in the air. When the runner moves from sea level to an elevation of 8,200 feet (Mexico City), the number of oxygen molecules in the lung will decrease nearly 30%. Under resting conditions there are few noticeable effects since the runner can simply increase his or her breathing to compensate for the lack of oxygen. With the increased demands of distance running, however, respiration becomes more limiting, and the ability to consume oxygen is reduced.

As illustrated in Figure 4-11, $\dot{V}O_2$max decreases roughly 3.2% for each 1,000-foot increase in altitude above 5,000 feet. Below 5,000 feet it is difficult to detect any decrement in performance or $\dot{V}O_2$max. Early studies demonstrated that the average time for a three-mile run at Mexico City was 8.5% slower than at sea level. In the mile run, performance decreased 3.6%. This means that a sea level time of 13 minutes for three miles would correspond to a 14 min:7s performance at an altitude of 7,500 feet.

In addition to the fewer number of oxygen molecules in the air, high altitude offers several other conditions which differ from sea level. Gas molecules in the air are further apart, so they offer less resistance as they move in and out of the lungs. Consequently, the runner's maximal breathing capacity is greater at alti-

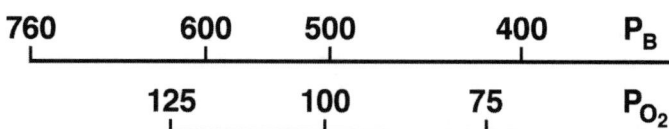

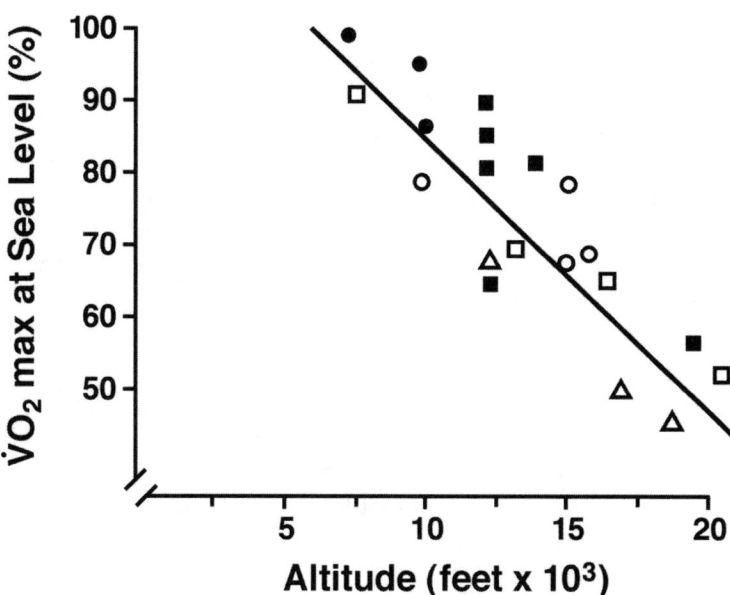

Figure 4-11. *The influence of altitude (barometric pressure, P_B, and oxygen tension, P_{O_2}) on maximal oxygen uptake, which decreased roughly 3.2 percent for each 1,000 feet increase in altitude above 5,000 feet.*

tude than at sea level. At the same time, there is less air at altitude to resist movement of the body. This is most noticeable in the sprint events, since air resistance changes with the wind velocity raised to the third power. Another consideration is the relatively cooler, drier air at altitude. Although this facilitates heat exchange, it also promotes respiratory water loss. As a result, many athletes lose weight abruptly through dehydration during the first few days at altitude, compounding their already reduced capacities for oxygen transport. Finally, solar radiation is more intense at altitude, which may cause sunburn and radiant heat gains during long runs.

The adaptations which result from endurance training at altitude are confined to: (1) an increase in breathing, (2) an increase in blood hemoglobin concentration, and (3) some small changes in muscle energy systems such as increased oxidative enzymes, myoglobin content, and capillarization. After a few days at high altitude runners are less able to tolerate lactate production, limiting their ability to perform repeated bouts of maximal anaerobic exercise.

Physiological adaptations to altitude are related to the duration of exposure. Since the rate of adaptation is not uniform for all physiological systems, full acclimatization to altitude may require several months.

Though there is some debate regarding the value of altitude training on performance at sea level, there is some suggestion that there might be some temporary benefits. Generally, however, evidence indicates the advantages are small. Studies in the 1960s and 70s indicated that there was little or no difference in the effect of hard endurance training at 7,500 feet and equivalently severe sea level training on $\dot{V}O_2$max values or two-mile performance times among runners who were already well conditioned. Training at altitude only improves performance at altitude. After twenty weeks of training at altitude the runners showed marked improvements in their performance at altitude.

There is no evidence to support the concept that breathing gases low in oxygen content while exercising for one to two hours per day will induce even a partial adaptation to altitude. It has, however, been demonstrated that this procedure may enhance the maximal exercise breathing capacity. Since most athletes cannot afford the time or expense involved in long stays at altitude, it is pertinent to consider the benefits for acclimatization of intermittent visits to altitude. Investigators have observed that alternating periods of training seven to 14 days at 7,500 feet with periods of five to 11 days at sea level was adequate for altitude acclimatization. Sea level stays of up to 11 days did not interfere with the usual adjustments to altitude as long as training was maintained.

Runners who wish to prepare for competition at moderate altitude must realize: (1) full adaptation may require several months, (2) work capacity must be reduced during the initial days at altitude, (3) the rate of acclimatization is unaffected by brief periods at sea level, (4) short exposure to gases containing reduced levels of oxygen will not stimulate adaptation to altitude, and (5) sea level performance is not improved by altitude training in runners who are already well-trained.

ALL THINGS CONSIDERED

Without a doubt, the most outstanding aspect of training is the ability of the body to adapt and become more tolerant of the physiological demands of repeated days and weeks of exercise. Improvements in blood circulation, oxygen delivery, energy production, and waste product removal make it possible for someone who could not run a single mile in 10 minutes before training to race in a marathon several minutes per mile faster. Though nearly all forms of regular aerobic exercise will improve one's endurance, the mode, frequency, and duration of training determine the degree of improvement in running performance.

Designing a training program for the distance runner is an art. The individual variations in human physiology, anatomy, and psychology make it impossible to design a single regimen that will meet the abilities and needs of all runners. Nevertheless, there are a number of factors in planning a training program that will help the runner reach his or her potential. These factors include the following:

1. **Specificity of training.** The physiological adaptations to training are closely related to the speed, distance, and mode of exercise performed during repeated days of exercise. Since there is little crossover from one type of exercise to another, the best way to prepare for distance competition is to run at speeds that develop the energy systems needed for racing. Non-specific exercises like cycling and swimming do little to prepare the individual for running.

2. **Balance work and rest.** The purpose of training is to stimulate the runner's anatomy and physiology to grow stronger during periods of rest and repair. Without adequate rest, the benefits of training cannot be fully realized.

3. **Hard days and easy days.** In addition to a need for complete rest, there must be some variation in the level of stress imposed during each training session. One or two days of hard training should be followed by a day or two of lighter intensity.

4. **Progression.** The body grows slowly and responds best to a gradual increase in training stress. Mileage and speed should be increased gradually over a period of several weeks and months. Although the progression of stress is always upward, weeks of hard training should always be followed by periods of markedly reduced effort.

5. **Mileage.** Although the number of calories burned during training seems to directly influence the degree of aerobic improvement, there is little value in running more than 60 to 100 miles per week. Mileage greater than that produces little, if any, improvement in the runner's performance or physiology. Lesser mileage allows greater opportunity for quality training.

6. **Hot and cold training.** Although circulation and sweating adjusts to exercise in the heat, there is little adaptation to cold weather running. Though heat acclimatization can be achieved after four to 12 days of training in a warm environment, the risk of heat injury is still the greatest single health threat to the runner.

7. **Altitude training.** Acclimatization to high altitude may take several months. Though running performances at altitude will improve with acclimation to altitude, training does not appear to improve a runner's performance at sea level.

CLASSIC AND SUGGESTED READINGS

Adams, W. C., L. M. Bernauer, D. B. Dill and J. B. Bomar. Effects of equivalent sea level and altitude training on $\dot{V}O_2$ and running performance. *J. Appl. Physiol.*, 39:262–266, 1975.

Brodal, P., F. Inger and L. Hermansen. Capillary supply of skeletal muscle fibers in untrained and endurance-trained men. *Am. J. Physiol.*, 232:H705–H712, 1977.

Buick, F. J., N. Gledhill, A. B. Froese and E. C. Spriet. Double blind study of blood boosting in highly trained runners. *Med. Sci. Sports*, 10:49, 1978.

Costill, D.L. What research tells the coach about distance running. *Am. Assoc. Health, Phys. Ed., Recreation,* 45–46, 1968.

Costill, D. L. and B. Saltin. Muscle glycogen and electrolytes following exercise and thermal dehydration. *Metabolic Adaptations to Prolonged Physical Exercise,* 352–360. Basel, Switzerland: Birkhauser Verlag, 1975.

Costill, D. L., E. F. Coyle, W. F. Fink, G. R. Lesmes and F. A. Witzmann. Adaptations in skeletal muscle following strength training. *J. Appl. Physiol.*, 46:96–99, 1979.

Costill, D. L., J. Daniels, W. Evans, W. Fink, G. Krahenbuhl and B. Saltin. Skeletal muscle enzymes and fiber composition in male and female track athletes. *J. Appl. Physiol.*, 40:149–154, 1976.

Costill, D. L., R. Cote, T. Miller and S. Wynder. Water and electrolyte replacement during repeated days of work in the heat. *Aviat. Space Environ. Med.*, 46;795–800, 1975.

Costill, D. L., W. Fink and M. Pollock. Muscle fiber composition and enzyme activities of elite distance runners. *Med. Sci. Sports,* 8:96–100, 1976.

Daniels, J. and N. Oldridge. The effects of alternate exposure to altitude and sea level on world-class middle-distance runners. *Med. Sci. Sports,* 2:107–112, 1970.

Ekblom, B., A. N. Goldbarg and B. Gullbring. Response to exercise after blood loss and reinfusion. *J. Appl. Physiol.*, 33:275–280, 1972.

Eriksson, B. O., P. D. Gollnick and B. Saltin. Muscle metabolism and enzyme activities after training in boys 11–13 years old. *Acta Physiol. Scand.*, 87:231–239, 1972.

Fox, E., R. Bartels, C. Billings, R. O'Brien, R. Bason and D. Mathews. Frequency and duration of interval training programs and changes in aerobic power. *J. Appl. Physiol.*, 38:481–484, 1975.

Fox, E. L., R. L. Bartels, C. E. Billings, D. K. Matthews, R. Bason and W. M. Webb. Intensity and distance of interval training programs and changes in aerobic power. *Med. Sci. Sports,* 5:18–22, 1973.

Grimby, G. and B. Saltin. A physiological analysis of still active middle-aged and old athletes. *Acta Med. Scand.*, 179:513–520, 1966.

Hermansen, L. and O. Vagge. Lactate disappearance and glycogen synthesis in human muscle after maximal exercise. *Am. J. Physiol.*, 233:E422–E429, 1977.

Horvath, S. M., Acclimatization to extreme cold. *Amer. J. Physiol.*, 150:99–108, 1947.

Pollock, M. The quantification of endurance training programs. *Exercise and Sports Sciences Reviews,* 1:155–188, 1973.

Pollock, M. L., T. K. Cureton and L. Greninger. Effects of frequency of training on working capacity, cardiovascular function, and body composition of adult men. *Med. Sci. Sports,* 1:70–74, 1969.

Pugh, L. G. C. Oxygen uptake in track and treadmill running with observations on the effect of air resistance. *J. Physiol.,* 207:825–835, 1970.

Pugh, L. G. C. Athletes at altitude. *J. Physiol.,* 192:619 747, 1967.

Robinson, S. Training, acclimatization and heat tolerance. *Proceedings of the International Symposium on Physical Actlvity and CardiovasculaY Health,* October 11–13, 1966.

Shrubb, A. A. Long distance running. *Training for Athletes,* 46–53 London: Health and Strength, Ltd., 1904.

Strydom, N. B. Acclimatization to humid heat and the role of physical conditioning. *J. Appl. Physiol.,* 21:636–642, 1966.

Chapter 5
The Female Distance Runner

INTRODUCTION

Efforts to describe the unique characteristics of the female distance runner commonly focus on the differences between men and women. The basic physiological and performance characteristics of female runners are no different than those of men. The cellular mechanisms controlling most physiological and biochemical responses to exercise are the same for both sexes. There are, however, several interesting gender variations in the magnitude of these physiological responses.

The majority of the scientific reports on running physiology and adaptations to training come from men. A large part of the explanation for the skewed profile of men as compared to women is that women were not prominent in sports until recently. As a result there is a growing base of physiology and training information that is specific for women participating in sports such as distance running. This chapter will focus on some of the unique aspects of female physiology and how it may impact training and performance.

PERFORMANCE: A MATTER OF GENDER

Figure 5-1 compares the difference between men and women's average running speeds measured in minutes per mile for the World record holders at distances from one mile to a marathon. On the average, women ran 10% slower than their male counterparts, a difference of about 30 seconds per mile. In two of the events (20K and 30K) women were approximately 15% slower or 45–60 seconds per mile. These comparisons may be a bit distorted, since these distances (12.4 and 18.6 miles) are not heavily contested.

Nevertheless, even at 6.2 miles (10 kilometers) and 26.2 miles (the marathon), two of the most frequently raced distances, the difference between the men and women's records averaged 11.5% or 29 seconds per mile for the 10K and 9.5% or 30 seconds per mile for the marathon. Thus, it appears that the difference in performance between the sexes is independent of the distance being run. When the 10-kilometer records for 20- to 35-year-old runners are averaged, the difference between men and women is again about 10% or 30 seconds per mile.

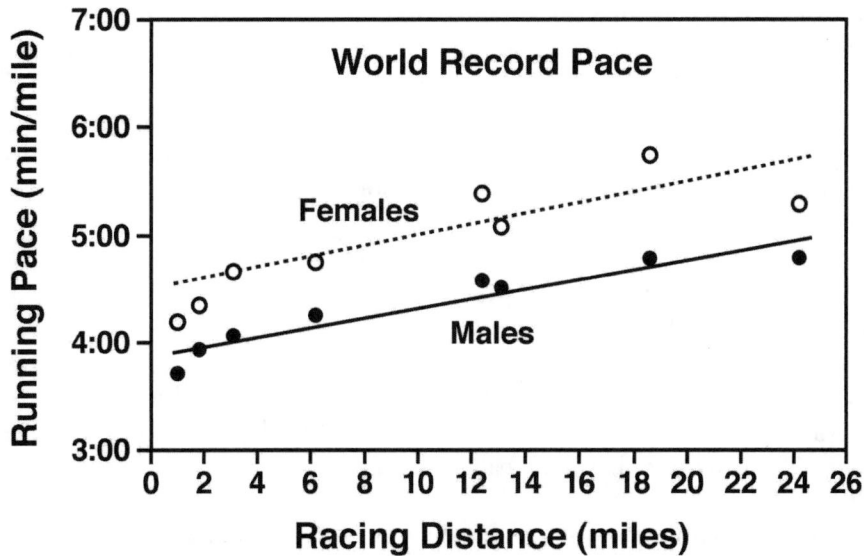

Figure 5-1. Shown is the world record running pace per mile for racing distances from one-mile through the marathon for males and females. Note that the average difference between men and women is maintained at approximately 11 to 12% independent of the distance run.

In 1985, the women's records indicated that they were 15% slower, or 40–45 seconds per mile slower compared to their male counterparts. This is most likely due to the increased number of female participants over the past several years. Since a greater number of females are now participating in distance running, the talent pool is larger. As a result, the records for women have improved at a greater rate than the men's records. Does this mean that women and men will be posting similar world records in another 30 years? Probably not. But these records do illustrate that the world records for female runners have closed to within 10% of the males.

Although it has been suggested that the performance differences between men and women are smaller at longer distances, the records do not agree. In the ultra-marathon events, the differences between men and women are even greater. Records ranging from 50km (31 mi) to 200 km (124 mi) are about 15% slower for women than men, an average difference in pace of 50 seconds to 2.5 minutes per mile.

Results from the 2001 Chicago marathon indicated that 28,648 people completed the marathon. Of those who did complete the marathon, 17,297 were men (60%) and 11,351 were women (40%). When averaging the top 10 male (2:10:38) and female (2:31:52) finishers from this race, the men ran 14% faster than the women. Comparing the top 10 male (2:34:09) and female (2:57:54) master competitors reveled that the men over 40 years of age were 13% faster than the women over 40 years old. It is interesting to note that the top male master runner (2:18:35) completed the marathon in almost the identical time as the top overall female (2:18:47). As noted above, the average of the top 10 female finishers and top 10 male master finishers posted nearly identical times. This data further illustrates that the top-level men run ~10–15% faster than women and this trend appears to continue into the master runners rank. Furthermore, the top-level female runners and top-level male master runners appear to perform similarly.

Of course there are many women who are faster than men. Many of the women who completed the Chicago marathon were faster than approximately half of the men who ran.

THE FEMALE TRIAD

The American College of Sports Medicine has addressed a clinically relevant condition that occurs in some female athletes who are engaged in heavy training. This condition has been called the female triad, or female athlete triad (Figure 5-2).

Women who train intensely and focus on weight loss may subject themselves to possible eating and menstruation disorders. Lower energy intake may result in chronic muscle fatigue which can negatively impact training, training adapta-

Figure 5-2. The female triad is sometimes observed in women who engage in heavy training and also have poor nutrition. This can often lead to physiological complications with the menstrual cycle and bone health.

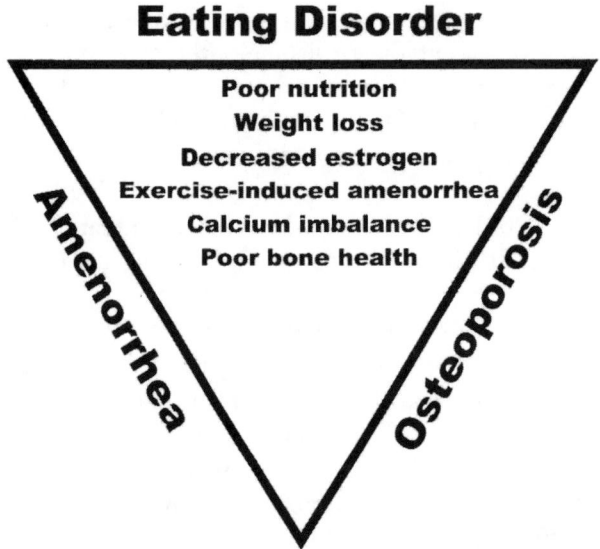

RUNNING: THE ATHLETE WITHIN

tions, and performance. The combination of hard training and loss of body fat may cause irregularities in menstrual cycle function (called amenorrhea). In severe cases, cessation of menstruation may exist for a period of several months. In fact, the cessation of menstruation is fairly common among endurance athletes who are training hard and competing. Most often, as the training subsides and proper nutrition is resumed, normal menstrual function returns.

Diagnosing the triad disorder is not easily understood and the causes are often debated among scientists and clinicians. However, many women who participate in running are likely to suffer from one of the triad's disorders, with the most common one being related to suboptimal eating and nutrient intake (under eating). The onset of amenorrhea is often the tell-tale sign or red flag of the disorder. Historically, amenorrhea has been associated with hard training and the price for athletic success. Of the female distance running population, it has been suggested that 25 to75% of women have experienced amenorrhea at some point in their running career. This is well above the national average of 5% in healthy females.

However, prolonged eating irregularities and amenorrhea may lead to more serious health conditions. As noted in Figure 5-3, a third component to the triad is bone health or osteoporosis. While it is difficult to determine the direct impact that run training, poor nutrition and the resulting amenorrhea have on bone health, regular functioning menstrual cycles have been positively linked to bone density. Thus, an extended period of amenorrhea (cessation of menstrual cycle or interspersed with regular cycles) may blunt normal bone growth resulting in lower bone density and more fragile bones. In particular, imbalances in calcium mediated through diet and amenorrhea have been implicated as one of the primary factors associated with a decrease in bone health. It has also been suggested that this may make bone more susceptible to fracture (i.e. stress fractures), which is often observed in the foot and the lower leg of female runners.

The hormone estrogen also influences the disturbance in calcium metabolism. Estrogen has a protective effect on the bone by promoting calcium absorption, reducing calcium loss in the urine, and decreasing bone remodeling. Any menstrual dysfunction suppresses estrogen levels; thereby decreasing the protective effect estrogen plays in maintaining healthy bones. Prolonged amenorrhea and the resulting disturbance in estrogen contributes to the loss in bone mass and increased risk for stress fractures. Even though normal menses may return, bone health may remain abnormal and result in suboptimal bone mass throughout adult life. This condition can predispose women to osteoporosis later in life.

While the female triad is not an exact science, the American College of Sports Medicine recommends that the treatment of the triad disorder begin within three months of the onset of amenorrhea. The successful treatment of the disorder can be mediated though psychological, nutritional, and training habits. More specifically, the following guidelines are recommended:

1. Reduce training volume and intensity by 20–25%.
2. Increase total caloric intake with a balanced diet.
3. Gradually begin to increase body weight.
4. Ingest daily calcium of 1200 mg.

By recognizing the symptoms of the female triad and properly treating the disorder with diet and reasonable training loads, health complications related to this disorder can be minimized and/or avoided.

BODY COMPOSITION

The fact that female runners have a higher percentage of body fat than males appears to account for some of the difference in running performances. As noted in Chapter 1, highly trained male distance runners have been reported to have 4 to 10% body fat. Female runners, on the other hand, have roughly 16% body fat, though some individual runners have less than 10%. Consequently, female runners carry an average of 9 to 12 pounds more body fat than the men. This additional weight requires the expenditure of more energy during running, thereby taxing the oxygen transport system to a greater relative degree when running at set (submaximal) speeds. Since the ability to maintain a fast pace during competition depends to a large degree on the fractional use of the aerobic capacity (amount of oxygen being consumed), a heavier runner would have to run a slower-pace per mile in order to expend the same relative effort.

This information might be taken to mean that every female runner should attempt to drop her body fat to 5 or 6%. Such a practice is neither necessary nor healthy. Though a number of the world's best female distance runners have body fat levels below 10%, many record holders have values above 14%. The body fat percentage of highly trained female runners is well below the 25% seen in the average untrained female. This difference is, for the most part, the result of heavy training rather than dieting.

Some runners may retain an atypical amount of body fat despite hard training. These individuals should be encouraged to diet during the less intense period of training and competition, since the stress of trying to run while consuming too few calories is certain to impair performance and may lead to a state of chronic fatigue (see Female Triad).

BONE HEALTH

In the previous discussion about the female triad, the balance among training, performance, nutrition, and overall health can be a delicate balance for the serious female athlete. Often times the desire for athletic success will cloud judgement when it comes to sound decisions regarding one's own health. This is further complicated by the fact that most people consider exercise as a positive form of stress. How could something as positive as exercise and fitness evolve into a bad thing? As with any physiological system in the human body, a disturbance in one facet of physiology can affect several other areas of physiology. This is the case during heavy run training and bone health, which is often measured by bone density and bone mineral content.

In general terms, exercise has been implicated as a positive stimulus for bone remodeling and stronger healthier bones. However, females are presented with a unique challenge for proper bone health, which is closely coupled to key female hormones in the body. In particular, hard run training can lead to hormone (estrogen) and ion (calcium) imbalances that can dramatically influence bone structure and formation.

Research in the area of women's health and female athletes with osteoporosis, has found that amenorrhea is linked with lower bone mineral density when compared to aged-matched normal menstruating athletes. These findings are summarized in Figure 5-3, which shows bone mineral densities (BMD) of the lumbar spine for regular menstruating women (NORMAL), athletic women with irregular menstrual cycles (IRREGULAR), and athletic women who have never had regular menstrual cycles (NEVER).

As can be seen in Figure 5-3, amenorrhea in the form of interspersed cycles and/or no menstrual cycles at all, profoundly impacts BMD. It also appears that the more severe the amenorrhea, the greater the loss in BMD. These data are

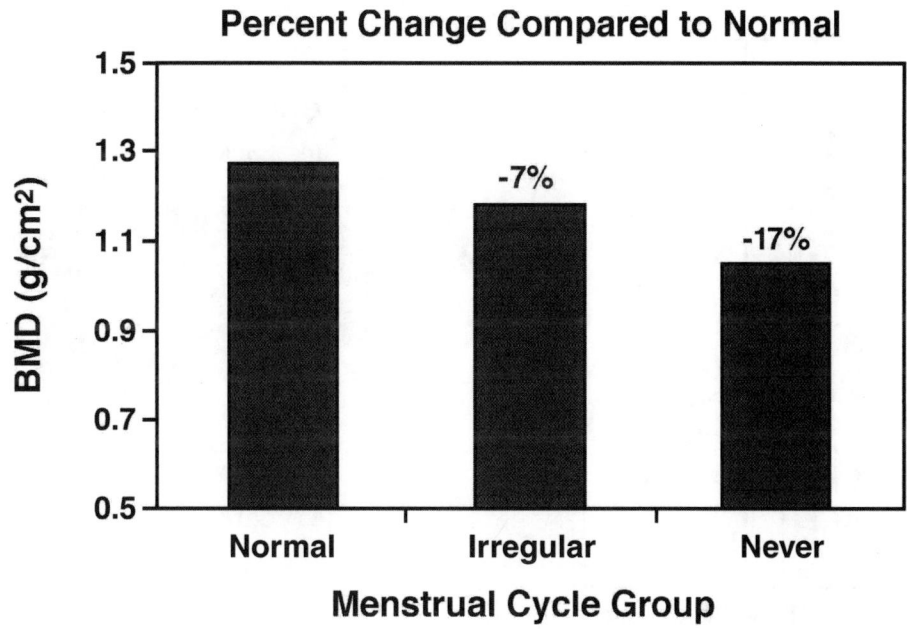

Figure 5-3. Shown is bone mineral density (BMD) in women who run with differing levels of menstrual function. Note that the women who have had prolonged amenorrhea have the greatest loss in BMD.

startling and highlight the importance of proper nutrition and menses for maintaining healthy bones.

Granted, not all female athletes will have low BMD, but females in heavy training who focus on weight loss and suffer from amenorrhea are particularly susceptible to low BMD. Research has clearly shown that poor nutrition and excessive training are linked to low BMD. Furthermore, this process appears to be chronic. That is, any bone health problems that are encountered early in life can lead to premature osteoporosis later in life. Some women who were amenorrheaic as teenagers and young adults have had osteoporosis complications as early as 30 years of age. The development of strong healthy bones is prominent in the first 3 decades of life, with peak bone mineral density occurring in females when they are 25 to 30 years old. Since most female athletes are engaged in heavy training between the ages of 15 and 30 years, they are particularly susceptible for low BMD and early onset osteoporosis.

Running posses a greater risk than most sports due to the loading nature on the skeleton while training. For example, a female runner weighing 120 pounds may have impact forces on the bone in excess of 500 pounds per stride. When the forces of running are coupled with amenorrhea and low bone density, the risk for stress fractures increases by 40–50%. Thus, the importance of BMD becomes rather clear when the impact nature of running is taken into account.

Figure 5-4 presents a bone scan from a healthy female runner. These scans are easy to conduct and harmless to the runner. In this example, the female runner is 27 years old and has been running for 10 years. She has a personal best of 2h:55min for the marathon and was running approximately 50 miles per week.

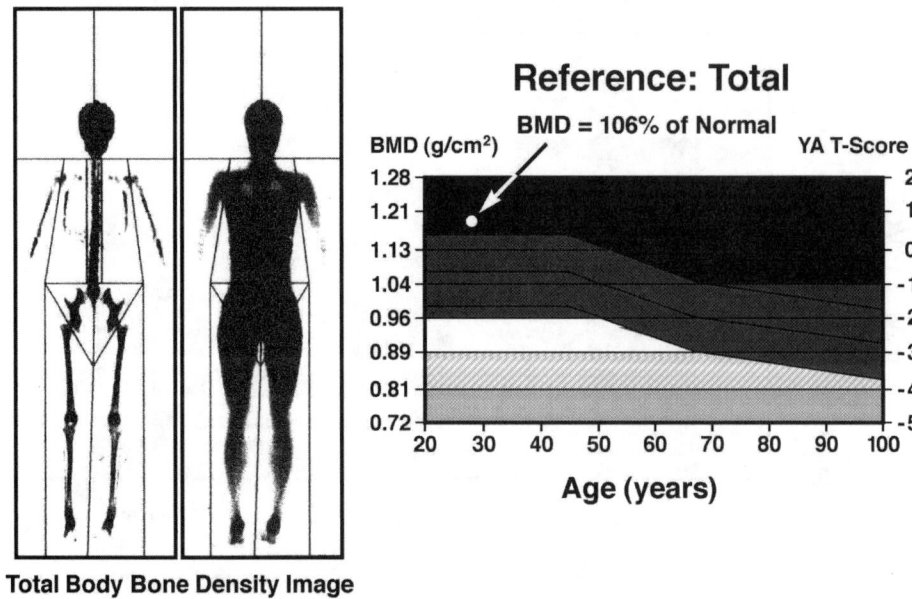

Figure 5-4. Shown is a total body bone scan from a healthy 27-year old runner with normal menstrual function. Her bone mineral density (BMD) was above normal (106%). Thus indicating that BMD can be maintained during hard run training with good nutrition and normal menstrual function.

Total Body Bone Density Image

As can be seen from the skeleton overview of this female runner, the bone mineral density and bone mineral content are within normal ranges. Her BMD was 106% compared to the general female population.

During the 10 years that she has been running she has had good eating habits and normal menstrual function for the last several years. Early in her running career she did experience mild bouts of amenorrhea. However, this can most likely be attributed to the initial increase in running volume and intensity coupled with inadequate nutrition.

MUSCLE COMPOSITION OF THE FEMALE RUNNER

In early studies with male and female track and field athletes we observed that there was little difference in the muscle fiber composition between the sexes. Scandinavian investigators have reported that among men and women, the amount of slow-twitch fibers made up about half (52%) of the total fiber population, with fast-twitch fibers making up the other half (48%) for both sexes. There is substantial evidence suggesting that there is no difference between men and women with regard to the percentage of slow-twitch and fast-twitch fibers. Regardless of gender, elite distance runners have a predominance of slow-twitch fibers in their leg muscles, ranging from 60–80% of the leg muscles.

The only reported difference in skeletal muscle fibers between the sexes is found in the size of the slow- and fast-twitch muscle fibers. In general, men have larger muscle fibers than women. Table 5-1 shows the size (cross-sectional area (um^2)) of slow-twitch and fast-twitch muscle fibers from untrained men and women. Also shown are the fiber size from highly trained male and female distance runners.

In the untrained population the muscle fibers of the men are 20 to 25% larger than the women. The 20 to 25% difference among the men and women appears to be of the same magnitude for both the slow-and fast-twitch muscle

TABLE 5-1. Skeletal muscle fiber composition (percent; %) and fiber size (cross-sectional area; μm^2) from inactive and distance trained men and women.

Group	% Slow-Twitch	Slow-Twitch Fiber Size	% Fast-Twitch	Fast-Twitch Fiber Size
Untrained				
Men	52	8008	48	7850
Women	51	6079	49	6218
Distance Runners				
Men	81	6613	19	5642
Women	79	5993	21	5018

fibers. Interestingly, the size of the muscle fibers in the trained distance runners paints a different picture. As with the untrained men and women, the male runners' muscle fibers were larger than the female runners, but only by 8 to 10%. Thus, it appears that for distance runners there is not as great a gender difference in the size among the muscle fibers. Also worth noting was that the untrained men and women had larger fibers than the runners. Little difference was found among the women; however the male distance runners' fibers were 15 to 25% smaller than the untrained men. The most likely explanation for this difference may be related to the impact distance running has on muscle fiber size. Since distance running is not a power sport and relies heavily upon aerobic conditioning and oxygen delivery, the smaller fibers are probably the result of metabolic adaptations from distance running. The smaller fibers make it easier to transport oxygen and fuels (carbohydrate and fat) from the blood to where they are needed in the muscle cell. Thus, the smaller diffusion distance allows for a more efficient working muscle cell for aerobic metabolism, which successful distance running requires. When compared to the muscle fiber size of the untrained men and women in Table 5-1, it is readily apparent that endurance training has a strong influence on the size of the fibers in males and females.

Since strength and speed are determined in part by muscle mass, the combined size of the muscle fibers is important to the performance of both male and female runners. Here, men have a slight advantage. But there is no evidence to suggest that men have more muscle fibers than women. The fact that well-trained men have only a small advantage in muscle fiber areas and that both sexes appear to have similar leg muscle development suggests that there is no major difference in the number of fibers.

ENERGY SYSTEMS

Delivery of oxygen and fuels to the muscles and removal of waste depends, in part, on the number of operational capillaries around each muscle fiber. Female runners have about 4.9 capillaries around each fiber, and male runners have about 5.6 capillaries per muscle fiber. This does not put the female runner at a disadvantage. Since the function of the capillaries is to allow for diffusion of chemicals in and out of the muscle cells, the size of the area served by each capillary is more important than the number of capillaries. Female runners have somewhat smaller muscle fibers, so the volume of muscle that must be served by each capillary is smaller in women than in men. This means that the exchange of materials between the muscle and the blood should be better in female than in male runners. There is no evidence, however, that this advantage has an impact on performance.

For both sexes there is a close relationship between a runner's $\dot{V}O_2$max and the average number of capillaries around each leg muscle fiber. Since both factors improve with endurance training, it appears that activity levels are more important than gender with regard to the number of capillaries in the muscle.

The capacity for aerobic energy production depends, in part, on the availability of mitochondria and their associated aerobic enzymes. Unfortunately, few data are available to compare the aerobic capacities of muscle in male and female distance runners. As can be seen in Table 5-2, male and female runners tend to have similar aerobic enzyme activities in their leg muscles.

Since aerobic enzymes give a good indication of how well a muscle can process and make aerobic energy from fat and carbohydrate, these are markers that are commonly used in exercise physiology to help gauge the aerobic potential of an individual. As can be seen, the distance runners' muscle is considerably more developed in terms of aerobic energy potential compared to the untrained men and women. While there are genetic limitations in each person's physiology, aerobic muscle enzymes can be improved with endurance training. Since the leg muscles of highly trained men and women have similar aerobic capacities, this factor alone cannot explain the differences in performance between elite men and women.

Some observers have suggested that women might be relatively better in longer events like the marathon because they could burn fat at a greater rate and generally have more fat to burn. This would enable the female runner to spare the use of muscle glycogen, thereby lowering her risk of running out of carbohydrate as a fuel source. We have refuted this theory by measuring the fat-burning capacity of the muscles from highly trained men and women. Muscle samples revealed that the men had a significantly greater capacity to use fat than the women, though this fact seemed to have little effect on the body's choice of fuels during exercise. When asked to run for an hour at marathon pace, both sexes derived about 50% of their energy from the breakdown of fat (with the other 50% coming from carbohydrate). It would appear that there is little or no difference

TABLE 5-2. Skeletal muscle aerobic enzyme activities (reported in $\mu m \bullet g^{-1} \bullet min^{-1}$) from inactive and distance run trained men and women.

Group	Succinate Dehydrogenase	Malate Dehydrogenase	Carnitine Palmityl Transferase
Untrained			
Men	7.6	48	0.7
Women	8.2	50	0.7
Distance Runners			
Men	17.7	71	1.0
Women	12.2°	72	0.8

° denotes difference between men and women.

in fat use or performance of highly trained men and women who have similar $\dot{V}O_2$max values and training backgrounds.

OXYGEN TRANSPORT

The best single determinant for distance running success is the capacity to consume, transport, and use oxygen. Elite female runners have somewhat lower $\dot{V}O_2$max values than top-level male runners. As noted earlier, the difference in performance between male and female distance running records is approximately 10%. Table 5-3 offers a comparison of $\dot{V}O_2$max and selected circulatory measurements for men and women. It is interesting to note that on the average, $\dot{V}O_2$max values for highly trained male and female runners differ by 20 to 25%. Since women have 6 to 8% more body fat than men, $\dot{V}O_2$max values for male and female runners differ by only 8 to 9% when calculated per kilogram of lean body weight.

Although both maximum stroke volume and maximum heart volume contribute to maximum volume of blood that can be pumped by the heart per minute, the size of the heart also appears to play a major role in determining the heart's pumping capacity. As noted in Table 5-3, the heart volume (HV) for men and women differs by 140 to 225 milliliters. Of course, heart size is somewhat related to an individual's body size. Measurements of heart volume per kilogram of body weight indicate that the male and female runners shown in Table 5-3 have about the same relative heart volume of 12.3 to 12.7 milliliters per kilogram of body weight. In other research, however, elite male distance runners have been reported to have an average heart volume of 16.4 milliliters per kilogram of body weight, meaning that highly trained men have hearts that are nearly 33% larger than elite female runners. It appears that a major part of the aerobic advantage

TABLE 5-3. Cardiovascular characteristics of men and women who are untrained and distance run trained.

Subjects	$\dot{V}O_2$max	HRmax	SVmax	Qmax	Heart Volume	Blood Volume
Untrained						
Men	48	192	109	21	785	5.25
Women	40	198	81	16	560	4.07
Distance Runners						
Men	70	187	144	27	930	6.58
Women	59	193	119	23	790	5.67

$\dot{V}O_2$max = maximal oxygen uptake (ml/kg/min); HRmax = maximal heart rate (beats/min); SVmax = Maximal Stroke Volume (ml/beat); Qmax = maximal cardiac output (liters/min); Heart volume (milliliters); Blood volume (liters).

held by male runners can be attributed to larger heart volume and its influence on the maximum volume of blood that can be pumped by the heart per minute.

Unfortunately, many of the comparative studies of male and female runners have used elite performers of each sex. Although such comparisons help us to understand the physiological basis for sex differences in running performance, there are few studies that have directly compared the physiological characteristics of men and women who have performed equally in distance running competition.

Recently, performance-matched female and male runners were studied to compare their physiological characteristics and responses during exercise. These men and women had similar training programs and performed equally well in a 15-mile race. In the laboratory, their physiological performances during submaximal and maximal treadmill running were also quite similar (Table 5-4).

The two groups shown in Table 5-4 used the same amount of oxygen during submaximal running, demonstrating that they had approximately the same running efficiency. The only notable difference between the men and women during exercise was a higher heart rate in females during the submaximal run, reflecting a smaller stroke volume. However, similar $\dot{V}O_2$ utilization during the submaximal run indicates that the men and women had a similar cardiac output (blood pumping from the heart per minute). Thus, the men and women had manipulated the heart rate and stroke volume to achieve nearly identical cardiac outputs and oxygen consumption during the submaximal effort. This is a common occurrence among athletes of both sexes. But typically, the better per-

TABLE 5-4. Physiological responses for maximal and submaximal treadmill running for performance matched male and female distance runners. Blood measurements shown were obtained from a resting sample.

Measurement	Females	Males
Maximal Run		
$\dot{V}O_2$max (ml/kg/min)	55	55
Heart Rate (beats/min)	186	189
Blood Lactate (mmol/l)	7.6	8.8
Submaximal Run (8 min/mile)		
$\dot{V}O_2$ (ml/kg/min)	43	42
Heart Rate (beats/min)	178°	169
Resting Blood Analysis		
Hematocrit (%)	40.6°	43.9
Hemoglobin (g/100ml)	14.1°	15.7
2,3 DPG (μm/g)	14.2°	12.2

2,3 DPG = 2,3 Diphosphoglyceric acid
° denotes significant difference between women and men

former will have a lower heart rate and higher stroke volume for a given oxygen consumption.

As mentioned in Chapter 1, hemoglobin plays a key role in transporting oxygen. Consequently, it is interesting to note that the female runners described in Table 5-4 had lower hemoglobin concentrations than the males, despite the fact that there was no difference in $\dot{V}O_2$max values for the two groups. This would suggest that in order to transport the same amount of oxygen per unit of blood, the women must have some means of compensating for their lower hemoglobin concentration. The mechanisms underlying such compensation are not known, but 2,3 diphosphoglyceric acid, known to facilitate the unloading of oxygen at the muscle, has been shown to be higher in female runners (Table 5-4). Though this might enhance the delivery of oxygen, it is only one of the possible mechanisms that might compensate for lower hemoglobin concentrations in female runners.

IRON SUPPLEMENTATION

Iron is a critical component for oxygen transport in the body. Iron provides the backbone for the hemoglobin and myoglobin molecules. In fact, the majority of iron in the body is used to help form hemoglobin and myoglobin. Hemoglobin works to carry oxygen from the lungs to the working muscles, while myoglobin works to store and transfer oxygen once inside the muscle cell.

Females have been targeted as a population that may be at risk for low iron stores and may need dietary supplementation. Iron loss can occur in menstruating women, pregnant women, women who under eat, and women who eat a vegetarian diet. Thus, low iron levels may provide an additional burden for females due to various physiological features unique to women (menstrual cycle and pregnancy).

Should female athletes take an iron supplement? On the surface this may seem like a trivial question. However, taking too much absorbable iron can be toxic to the body. Even when iron supplements are taken, it is not easily incorporated to produce higher hemoglobin and myoglobin levels. For women who meet or exceed the recommended iron intake, iron supplementation does not increase hemoglobin or hematocrit levels in the body. In other words, there is no ergogenic benefit for additional iron intake in people who meet the recommended daily allowance.

The term sports anemia has been popularized over the last several years to describe the reduced hemoglobin level sometimes observed in athletic females (<12 g/dl). Females that are at risk for low iron stores should see a physician and get some nutritional counseling. Generally, it is recommended that women who want to avoid low iron stores should eat a well-balanced diet and carefully monitor their training.

STRENGTH AND SPEED

Although muscle strength is not considered a critical factor for distance running success, it may affect the runner's speed and running mechanics. For that reason, it is interesting to note that on average women have about one third less muscle strength than men. Research has demonstrated that when muscle strength is expressed in terms of total body weight or lean body weight, strength differences between the sexes are reduced.

Figure 5-5 shows the strength differences in leg extension (i.e. leg press) of young college men and women. From this data it appears that when corrected for lean body mass, there is no measurable difference in leg extension strength among men and women.

Recent studies have shown that men and women have similar leg strength when they perform maximal muscle contractions at relatively slow leg movements. At faster movements, however, men were significantly stronger than women. The reason for these differences in leg strength at slow and fast speeds is unknown, although these results suggest that men and women recruit different muscle fibers or that there is some difference in the contractile properties of their muscle fibers. Since we do not know the fiber composition of the subjects used in any of these strength studies, we cannot attribute the differences in upper and lower body strength to variations in the number of fast- or slow-twitch fibers.

Previous studies have made it clear that the potential for force development is the same in muscle samples taken from both men and women. As can be seen

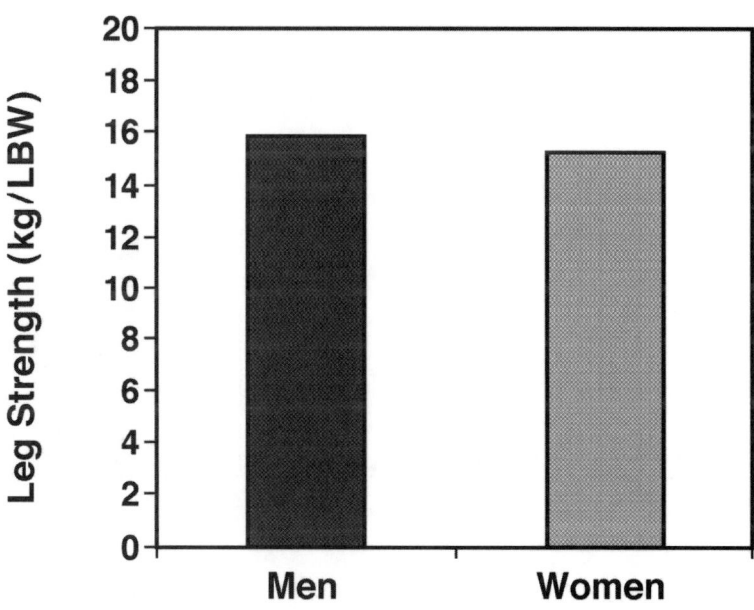

Figure 5-5. *Leg strength (men/women) corrected for muscle size. Although women typically have smaller muscles than men, their strength is the same per unit size.*

in Figure 5-6, arm strength is closely related to the size of the muscle in both men and women. The strength of a single muscle fiber is unaffected by the individual's sex. The major determinant of overall strength is the size of the muscle. The larger muscle has more contractile filaments (actin and myosin) and therefore possesses greater potential for force development when it is activated.

Physiologists have repeatedly demonstrated that strength training produces greater muscle hypertrophy in men than in women. In fact, strength training in females seldom produces the muscle bulk commonly seen in men. Muscular hypertrophy is regulated mainly by the hormone testosterone, which is approximately 10 times higher in the blood of men than in women.

Since both men and women seem to have approximately the same leg strength per unit of lean body weight, the differences between men and women in distance running performances cannot be explained by a lack of leg strength in the females. Specific leg strength and cross-sectional muscle mass, however, have not been measured in female and male distance runners.

Since sprint runs of 100 and 200 meters require maximal force development in both the upper and lower body, men tend to have a 9 to 10% performance advantage in these events. Total body strength may also play a role in determining one's running speed during distance running, though this point remains to be clarified.

Although men and women have similar leg strength, it is difficult to understand why there is such a marked disparity in upper body muscle development

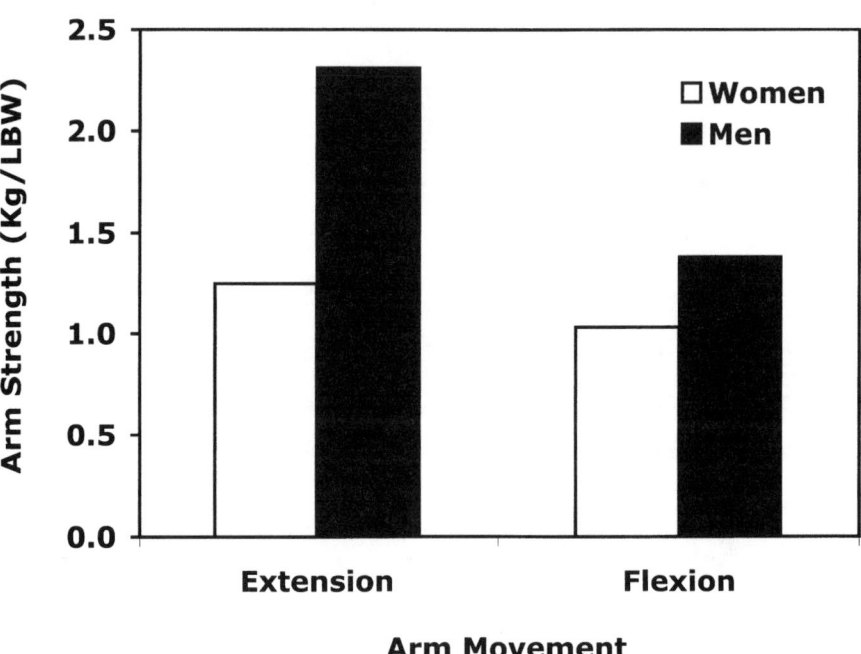

Figure 5-6. Arm strength (men/women) corrected for muscle size. For arm extension it appears that men may have a greater strength per unit of muscle mass.

RUNNING: THE ATHLETE WITHIN

between the sexes. One might anticipate that the hormonal mechanisms responsible for muscle development in the legs would have the same influence on the arm muscles. Apparently this is not the case, which makes it difficult to understand what processes could control the differentiation of fiber growth and muscle hypertrophy in the arms and legs. The regulators are most likely associated with the hormonal characteristics of the sexes. In particular the genetic differences in testosterone levels in the body appear to play a key role in muscle development. Given that men have about 10-fold higher levels of testosterone than women, this may be one of the primary reasons that men have a much greater potential for muscle development and building muscle mass.

HEAT TOLERANCE

Heat stress offers the greatest single threat to the health of the distance runner. Although training and repeated days of heat exposure provide some tolerance to the heat, there are marked individual variations in the ability to dissipate body heat. While women have significantly more body fat and appear to produce smaller amounts of sweat during exercise than men, they do not run a higher risk of heat injury during distance running. The number of heat-related problems in women during running in hot weather is no greater for women than it is for men.

Few studies have been conducted to assess the tolerance of endurance-trained women to long-term submaximal exercise in the heat. In many cases the women used in studies on heat stress were relatively sedentary, with significantly lower aerobic capacities than the men to whom they were compared. Under these conditions, when both sexes were required to exercise at the same absolute intensity, women had higher heart rates and internal body temperatures.

Since male and female distance runners use about the same percentage of their maximal oxygen uptakes during distance races, it is more appropriate to examine heat tolerance when the subjects are running at the same percent $\dot{V}O_2$max. When the exercise task is matched to the runner's aerobic capacity, the physiological responses to heat stress are similar for both men and women. The only notable differences in their responses to the heat are that men tend to produce more sweat and begin sweating sooner than women. Although this may be an advantage during exercise in a hot, dry environment, it also subjects men to a greater rate of dehydration. Despite their lower rates of sweating, trained women are able to dissipate body heat and become acclimatized equally as well as men.

TRAINABILITY

Despite differences in aerobic endurance and muscle strength, men and women appear to adapt to training in much the same way. Females benefit from training just as males do. When men and women train together, their adaptations are nearly identical. During regular continuous and interval training, men have been shown to increase their $\dot{V}O_2$max values 15%, while women had a 14% improvement. Heart rate and blood lactate responses during maximal and submaximal exercise did not differ between the sexes or as a result of the style of training.

Male and female cadets at the U S. Military Academy were studied during their initial training indoctrination. The women improved their aerobic capacity by 8%, whereas the men showed only a 2% increase in $\dot{V}O_2$max values. The smaller improvement in the men was attributed to the fact that they were in better condition than the women at the beginning of the training program (59 ml/kg × min). There have been some suggestions that the mechanisms underlying the improvements in $\dot{V}O_2$max with training may differ between the sexes. When women are trained at relatively high intensities of 70 and 100% $\dot{V}O_2$max, however, the cardiovascular and respiratory adjustments are similar to those of men.

EXERCISE DURING PREGNANCY

Should females continue to run during pregnancy? There is a growing body of research to support run training and competition while pregnant. Especially in the early stages, or first trimester of pregnancy. In fact, the American College of Obstetricians and Gynecologists recommends regular physical activity during pregnancy. There are, however, several physiological considerations that should be taken into account for pregnant females who want to run. In particular, women should be aware of how being pregnant will affect the physiological responses to running, adaptations to training, performance, and how nutritional demands will change. Nonetheless, the current information available does not suggest that there is an increased risk to women who regularly exercise as long as they follow some practical cautionary measures.

Physiological Responses to Exercise During Pregnancy

One of the major changes that occur with pregnancy is the formation of new tissue for the fetus and the resulting 15 to 20% increase in metabolic rate. This leads to a series of changes in body composition and physiological function in women who are pregnant. While most people may associate pregnancy as a negative for female physiology, there are several positive adaptations that occur to the female body.

Other than a bigger stomach, one of the more notable aspects of being pregnant is the increased cardiovascular demand on the female to properly oxygenate the fetus. Research has shown that both blood volume and cardiac output (total amount of blood pumped out of the heart per minute) increase during pregnancy. Shortly after conception, there are dramatic changes in hormone balance that stimulates salt and water retention, thereby increasing blood volume. The increased blood volume increases stroke volume with varied affects on heart rate. The increased blood volume and resulting improvements in cardiac output improves the amount of oxygen that can be delivered. This, in turn, causes the heart rate to drop slightly at rest and during mild exercise. As a result, the cardiovascular system becomes more efficient at delivering oxygen to the working muscles during exercise.

Maximal breathing capacity is unchanged during pregnancy. The fetus causes a change in the rib-cage configuration that may cause a slight increase in vital capacity of the lungs. However, there is a rise in the resting breathing volume (called tidal volume). This increase in tidal volume has little effect on the transport of oxygen into the body and transport of carbon dioxide out of the body. This is due to the small changes in gas diffusion gradients and enhanced gas exchange at the tissue level. Female runners who are pregnant can expect little reduction in ventilation and $\dot{V}O_2$max. In fact, research has shown that $\dot{V}O_2$max may be enhanced slightly when run training is continued during pregnancy.

Thermoregulation during pregnancy has been a concern for runners due to the potential harmful affects that overheating may have on the fetus. During pregnancy resting core temperature drops due to greater heat dissipation. This also carries over to exercise. During exercise, research has shown that thermal stress is reduced while pregnant. This "cooling effect" is primarily related to the increased blood volume and skin blood flow which assists in carrying heat away from the core (and thus the fetus) to the skin to dissipate in the environment. This is further assisted by the fact that the blood vessels are more easily dilated to carry more blood due to hormonal changes that occur during pregnancy. Another factor is the increasing body weight that acts as a thermal buffer by increasing the amount of heat necessary to increase overall body temperature. These data suggest that when training is continued during pregnancy, the thermoregulatory adaptations appear to offset the possibility of excessive thermal load for both the mother and the fetus. However, pregnant runners should use caution and sound judgment. Running in excessive heat can still lead to intolerable heat stress that can be hazardous for the mother and fetus.

Probably the most notable feature of pregnancy is weight gain. While an increase in body weight cannot be avoided during pregnancy, research has shown that continued aerobic exercise can limit weight gain. Figure 5-7 shows the weight gain in early and late pregnancy in a group of female runners and a group of women who did not exercise while pregnant.

As can be seen from Figure 5-7, the majority of the weight-gain between the runners and non-exercisers occurred during the last phases of pregnancy. Overall, the non-exercisers gained about 10 more pounds than the runners. This could be advantageous during pregnancy since there would be less body weight

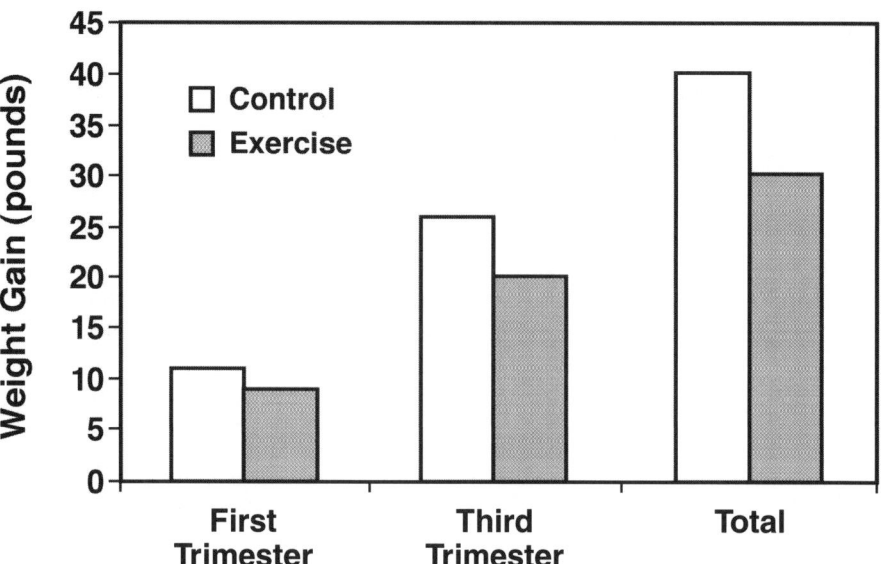

Figure 5-7. Shown are body weights for women who exercised and women who did not exercise during pregnancy. In both cases weight gain can be expected. However, in the women who exercised the total amount of weight gain during pregnancy can be expected to be less than if they did not exercise at all.

to carry during training and also after the pregnancy in returning to pre-pregnancy body weight.

Another area of concern is possible alteration in the metabolism of fuels (fat and carbohydrate) during pregnancy. Research in this area is lacking, but there are some studies that suggest that fuel metabolism may be altered during pregnancy. In particular, there appears to be a slight drop in available glucose with an increase in the amount of circulating free fatty acids during exercise. It is believed that the increased nutritional demands by the fetus take priority for glucose metabolism. As a result, the mother has to rely more upon fat as a substrate and internal carbohydrate stores (i.e. muscle glycogen) during running. This becomes even more pronounced as the gestation period progresses. However, regular sustained exercise does not appear to pose any nutritional danger for the fetus or the mother.

Training and Performance During Pregnancy

There does not appear to be any major physiological hurdles or identifiable risks that would prevent females from continuing to run and compete while pregnant. In fact, exercise prior to and during pregnancy is encouraged to help the physiological conditioning of the mother. Research suggests both the mother and the fetus should benefit from a regular fitness program such as running. A similar approach should be taken in developing and implementing a training program for pregnant women as if she were not pregnant. The basics of training and performance for expectant mothers really involve common sense and modification during pregnancy. As for modification of the training program, items to help protect the mother and fetus should be implemented. For example, it would not be wise to run outside on slippery winter days as to fall and injure the mother or fetus. Additionally, climbing Mt. Everest or running a marathon during the third trimester would not be advisable. Bottom line is to use some common sense and follow practical training guidelines while pregnant.

Anecdotally, most people would assume that performance would be compromised once pregnant. However, running performance may be enhanced during the early phases of pregnancy. As discussed earlier, there are several physiological changes that occur in the female following conception. Primarily the hormonal and cardiovascular shifts can be beneficial for performance. There is an increase in blood volume, which in turn improves cardiac output and delivery of oxygen to working muscles. Since there is little weight gain in the early phases of pregnancy, these cardiovascular enhancements may prove to be advantageous for running performance. There are anecdotal reports of females who have performed very well in the first trimester of pregnancy; however, solid research to substantiate these claims is lacking. Obviously, as the gestation period progresses, the additional weight gain will cause an increase in joint stress.

Nutritional Concerns

Little to no data exists to give exact nutritional recommendations to pregnant females. In general, there is concern that women who regularly engage in exercise during pregnancy need to increase their energy intake to ensure proper development of the fetus. For the pregnant female there are several aspects of metabolism to take into account. There is a large variation in resting metabolic rate, adaptation to the pregnancy, frequency of exercise, intensity of exercise, and duration of exercise will all impact nutritional demands. Thus, the general recommendation is to eat a well balanced diet and allow the normal increase in body weight to occur. In addition to monitoring dietary intake, normal physical check-ups of the mother and fetus will help ensure that the proper growth rate and development of the fetus is occurring.

Supplementation of various vitamins and minerals has been suggested, but not scientifically proven to be necessary during pregnancy. In particular, additional calcium, iron, and folic acid offer the most practical and basic micronutrients that should provide the female with additional levels of micronutrients that may be lacking, especially in vegetarians or other special diet populations.

Final Thoughts for Pregnant Women

Overall, female runners who become pregnant can and should continue to exercise. Moderate exercise appears to be beneficial for both mother and fetus during the gestation period. Recommendations include a practical common sense approach to training, competition, and nutritional intake. For healthy females, continued run training as part of a specific training program is reasonable.

SUMMARY

The information in this chapter provides the physiological basis for inherit differences among males and females. In general, females tend perform ~10% slower than their male counterparts. From the research that has been conducted, it appears that a large portion of this difference can be attributed to a smaller cardiovascular system and smaller muscles of the female athlete. For the female athlete, it is apparent that there are additional physiological challenges that include menses and pregnancy. However, if managed properly, females can continue to exercise without the risk to their own physiology or the development of the fetus. Lastly, females in heavy training should closely monitor their training and dietary habits to avoid potentially harmful side effects. With proper diet and awareness, women can train and compete at a high level without fear of physiological injury.

CLASSIC AND SUGGESTED READINGS

Asmussen E. Isometric muscle strength of adult men and women. *In: Communications from the testing and Observation Institute of the Danish Association for the Infantile Paralysis 11*, 1961.

Åstrand P-O. Human physical fitness with special reference to sex and age. *Physiol. Rev.* 36: 307–334, 1956.

Bar-or, D. Lamb and P. Clarkson. Exercise and the female — A life span approach. In: *Perspectives in Exercise Science and Sports Medicine*. Traverse City, MI: Cooper Publishing Group, 2001, p. 458.

Blair S.N., E. Horton, A.S. Leon, I.M. Lee, B.L. Drinkwater, R. K. Dishman, M. Mackey and M.L. Kienholz. Physical activity, nutrition, and chronic disease. *Med Sci Sports Exerc* 28: 335–349, 1996.

Brown C.H. and J.H. Wilmore. The effects of maximal resistance training on the strength and body composition of women athletes. *Med Sci Sports* 6: 174–177, 1974.

Clapp J.F., 3rd. A clinical approach to exercise during pregnancy. *Clin Sports Med* 13: 443–458, 1994.

Clapp J.F., 3rd and K.D. Little. The interaction between regular exercise and selected aspects of women's health. *Am J Obstet Gynecol* 173: 2–9, 1995.

Clapp J.F., 3rd and E. Capeless. Cardiovascular function before, during, and after the first and subsequent pregnancies. *Am J Cardiol* 80: 1469–1473, 1997.

Clapp J.F., 3rd. Exercise during pregnancy. A clinical update. *Clin Sports Med* 19: 273–286, 2000.

Clarkson P.M. Minerals: exercise performance and supplementation in athletes. *J Sports Sci* 9 Spec No: 91–116, 1991.

Clarkson P.M. and E.M. Haymes. Exercise and mineral status of athletes: calcium, magnesium, phosphorus, and iron. *Med Sci Sports Exerc* 27: 831–843, 1995.

Cohen J.S. and C.V. Gisolfi. Effects of interval training on work-heat tolerance of young women. *Med Sci Sports Exerc* 14: 46–52, 1982.

Costill D.L., G. Branam, D. Eddy and K. Sparks. Determinants of marathon running success. *Internationale Zeitschrift fur angewandte Physiologie* 29: 249–254, 1971.

Costill D.L., J. Daniels, W.J. Evans, W.J. Fink, G. Krahenbuhl and B. Saltin. Skeletal muscle enzymes and fiber composition in male and female track athletes. *Journal of Applied Physiology* 40: 149–154, 1976.

Creighton D.L., A.L. Morgan, D. Boardley and P.G. Brolinson. Weight-bearing exercise and markers of bone turnover in female athletes. *J Appl Physiol* 90: 565–570, 2001.

Daniels W.L., D.M. Kowal, J.A. Vogel and R.M. Stauffer. Physiological effects of a military training program on male and female cadets. *Aviat Space Environ Med* 50: 562–566, 1979.

Daniels W.L., J.E. Wright, D.S. Sharp, D.M. Kowal, R.P. Mello and R.S. Stauffer. The effect of two years' training on aerobic power and muscle strength in male and female cadets. *Aviat Space Environ Med* 53: 117–121, 1982.

Dook J.E., C. James, N.K. Henderson and R.I. Price. Exercise and bone mineral density in mature female athletes. *Med Sci Sports Exerc* 29: 291–296, 1997.

Drinkwater B.L., I.C. Kupprat, J.E. Denton and S.M. Horvath. Heat tolerance of female distance runners. *Ann N Y Acad Sci* 301: 777–792, 1977.

Drinkwater B.L. Women and exercise: physiological aspects. *Exerc Sport Sci Rev* 12: 21–51, 1984.

Drinkwater B.L., K. Nilson, C.H. Chesnut, W.J. Bremner, S. Shainholtz and M.B. Southworth. Bone mineral content of amenorrheic and eumenorrheic athletes. *N Engl J Med* 311: 277–281, 1984.

Drinkwater B.L., K. Nilson, S. Ott and C.H. Chesnut. Bone mineral density after resumption of menses in amenorrheic athletes. *JAMA* 256: 380–382, 1986.

Drinkwater B.L. Physical exercise and bone health. *J Am Med Womens Assoc* 45: 91–97, 1990.

Drinkwater B.L., B. Bruemner and C.H. Chesnut. Menstrual history as a determinant of current bone density in young athletes. *JAMA* 263: 545–548, 1990.

Drinkwater B.L. and C.H. Chesnut. Bone density changes during pregnancy and lactation in active women: a longitudinal study. *Bone Miner* 14: 153–160, 1991.

Ernst E. Exercise for female osteoporosis. A systematic review of randomised clinical trials. *Sports Med* 25: 359–368, 1998.

Gisolfi C.V. and J.S. Cohen. Relationships among training, heat acclimation, and heat tolerance in men and women: the controversy revisited. *Med Sci Sports* 11: 56–59, 1979.

Hatoum N., J.F. Clapp, M.R. Newman, N. Dajani and S.B. Amini. Effects of maternal exercise on fetal activity in late gestation. *J Matern Fetal Med* 6: 134–139, 1997.

Keen A.D. and B.L. Drinkwater. Irreversible bone loss in former amenorrheic athletes. *Osteoporos Int* 7: 311–315, 1997.

Kilbom A. Effect on women of physical training with low intensities. *Scand J Clin Lab Invest* 28: 345–352, 1971.

Kilbom A. and I. Astrand. Physical training with submaximal intensities in women. II. Effect on cardiac output. *Scand J Clin Lab Invest* 28: 163–175, 1971.

Kilbom A. Physical training in women. *Scand J Clin Lab Invest Suppl* 119: 1–34, 1971.

Otis C.L., B. Drinkwater, M. Johnson, A. Loucks and J.H. Wilmore. American College of Sports Medicine position stand. The Female Athlete Triad. *Med Sci Sports Exerc* 29: i–ix, 1997.

Rajaram S., C.M. Weaver, R.M. Lyle, D.A. Sedlock, B. Martin, T.J. Templin, J.L. Beard and S.S. Percival. Effects of long-term moderate exercise on iron status in young women. *Med Sci Sports Exerc* 27: 1105–1110, 1995.

Rencken M.L., C.H. Chesnut and B.L. Drinkwater. Bone density at multiple skeletal sites in amenorrheic athletes. *JAMA* 276: 238–240, 1996.

Saltin B. and P-O. Astrand. Maximal oxygen uptake in athletes. *J Appl Physiol* 23: 353–358, 1967.

Seals D.R., J.M. Hagberg, B.F. Hurley, A.A. Ehsani and J.O. Holloszy. Endurance training in older men and women I. Cardiovascular responses to exercise. *Journal of Applied Physiology* 57: 1024–1029, 1984.

Speechly D.P., S.R. Taylor and G.G. Rogers. Differences in ultra-endurance exercise in performance-matched male and female runners. *Med Sci Sports Exerc* 28: 359–365, 1996.

Warren M.P. and N.E. Perlroth. The effects of intense exercise on the female reproductive system. *J Endocrinol* 170: 3–11, 2001.

Wilmore J.H. and C.H. Brown. Physiological profiles of women distance runners. *Med Sci Sports* 6: 178–181, 1974.

Wilmore J.H., C.H. Brown and J.A. Davis. Body physique and composition of the female distance runner. *Ann N Y Acad Sci* 301: 764–776, 1977.

Yeager K.K., R. Agostini, A. Nattiv and B. Drinkwater. The female athlete triad: disordered eating, amenorrhea, osteoporosis. *Med Sci Sports Exerc* 25: 775–777, 1993.

Chapter 6
The Aging Distance Runner: Use It Or Lose It!

INTRODUCTION

For most athletes who exercise and compete, performing at their best is the ultimate goal. Despite hard training, good nutrition, or inherent talent, all runners can expect a gradual decay in peak running performance with aging. Generally, after you reach your late thirties or early forties you are unlikely to experience a lifetime best performance. The decline in running performance is even more pronounced as you enter the fifth decade of life and beyond. The bottom line is that aging takes it toll, even on the best and most dedicated runners.

The master athlete, also referred to as a veteran runner, constitutes a large portion of the participants in today's local and national competitions. This increased participation of older runners has raised considerable interest in the physiological changes that occur in our bodies with aging. This chapter will offer some insights that help explain the physiological and performance changes that occur throughout life.

PERFORMANCE: AGE 40 AND BEYOND

Most world records in running are set by adults in their middle-to-late twenties, though some individuals have achieved world level performances well beyond that age. Since master running records generally start at age 40, this is a logical age comparison since most runners use the 40-year mark to re-dedicate themselves to achieve peak performance. In Table 6-1 and 6-2 the world records and master world records for men and women's running events ranging from 100 meters to the marathon are shown. These records clearly illustrate that there is a decline in performance despite a dedicated training plan in highly motivated runners. On average, a 4 to 8% decline in performance can be expected by the forth decade of life. However, worth noting is that the times established by the 40 year old master athlete are quite impressive over all distances.

Perhaps the most exceptional records are the master marathon records for males and females. Mohamed Ezzher ran a 2h:10min:32s marathon in April 2001. This represents about 11 seconds slower per mile (4min:58s/mile pace)

Historical Note
Dr. Jack Daniels has, perhaps, tested more distance runners than any other sports scientist. When asked about his most interesting findings he stated: "In the summer of 1968 we tested 26 Olympic male distance runners. Their average maximal oxygen uptake was 77.8 ml × kg × min. The same guys (all 26) 25 years later averaged 57.5 max/kg × min."

TABLE 6-1. Men's World Records and Master World Records for the 100 meters, mile, 10,000 meters and the marathon. For each event, the first line represents the world best, while the second line represents the masters' world best.

Event	Performance	% Decline	Name	Age	Date
100m	9.79		Maurice Green	24	16-Jun-99
	10.60	−8.3	Eddie Hart	40	16-Sep-89
Mile	3:43.13		Hicham El Guerrouj	24	7-Jul-99
	3:58.13	−6.7	Eamonn Coghlan	41	20-Feb-94
10,000m	26:22.75		Haile Gebrselassie	25	1-Jun-98
	28:30.88	−8.1	Martti Vainio	40	25-Jun-91
Marathon	2:05.38		Khalid Khannouchi	27	14-Apr-02
	2:10.32	−3.9	Mohamed Ezzher	40	8-Apr-01

TABLE 6-2. Women's World Records and Master World Records for the 100 meters, mile, 10,000 meters and the marathon. For each event, the first line represents the world best, while the second line represents the masters' world best.

Event	Performance	% Decline	Name	Age	Date
100m	10.49		Florence Griffith Joyner	29	16-Jul-88
	11.99	−14.3	Zdenke Mosika	40	20-Jul-97
Mile	4:12.56		Svelana Masterkova	28	23-Aug-96
	4:23.78	−4.4	Yekatarina Podkopayeva	40	9-Jun-93
10,000m	29:31.78		Wang Junxia	20	8-Sep-93
	32:12.07	−8.7	Nicole Leveque	42	13-Aug-94
Marathon	2:18.47		Catherine Ndereba	25	7-Oct-01
	2:26.51	−4.4	Prescilla Welch	40	10-May-87

compared to the 2h:05min:42s (4min:47s/mile pace) world best set by Khalid Khannouchi in October of 1999. Only a few talented runners in the world, especially a 40 year old, could hope to run a marathon of this caliber. Interestingly, the female marathon record shows a similar pattern, with the master world record only 6 minutes slower than the world marathon record. This clearly shows that older athletes are capable of outstanding, world-class performances.

Another topic of interest to runners is the rate of decline in performance with age. The general data on aging and strength suggests that explosive power type movements are lost first, or at a faster rate compared to normal physical activities. It has been suggested that this is related to a selective loss of fast-twitch (power-type) muscle fibers as we age (see Chapter 3 and the following). However, these studies are limited and have not involved people who have led active lifestyles. When examining the record times for events from the 100-meter dash and the marathon it appears that there is a similar drop-off in performance (Figure 6-1 and 6-2).

Shown in Figure 6-1 and 6-2 is the percent decline in performance for the one-mile and the marathon. The drop-off in performance for these two events is compared to the world record for each event. For example, for the mile, there is about a 7% decline in performance for a 40 year old compared to the world record (3min:43s compared to 3min:58s). By age 65, the best mile time is 33% slower than the world record. In both events, there is a rather modest decline (about 45%) in performance from age 20 to age 70. Beyond age 70 there is an

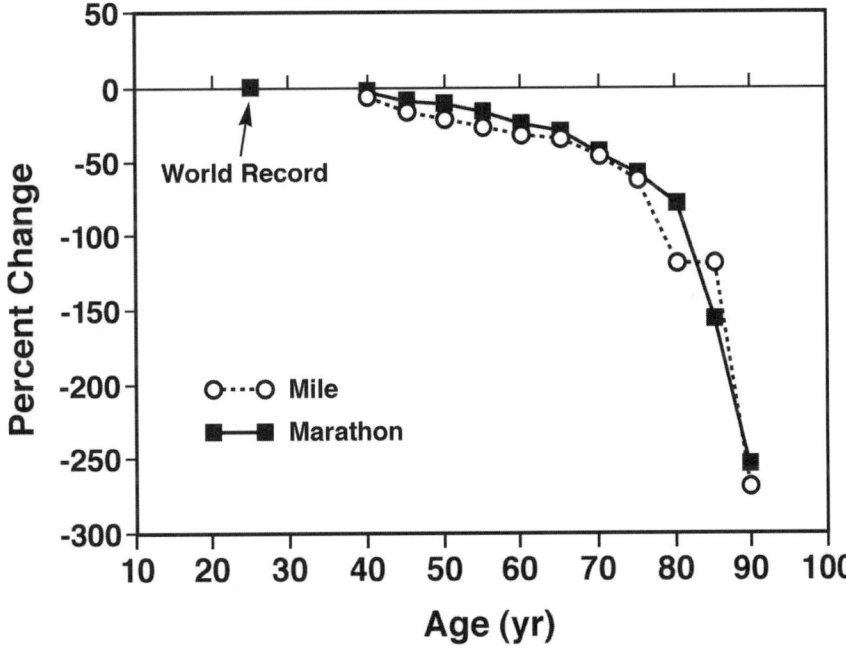

Figure 6-1. Men's decline in performance in the 100 meters (sprint event) and marathon (endurance event) with age. Note the rapid decline in performance after age 70 years. Also note the similarities in the rate of decline in performance between the sprint and endurance events.

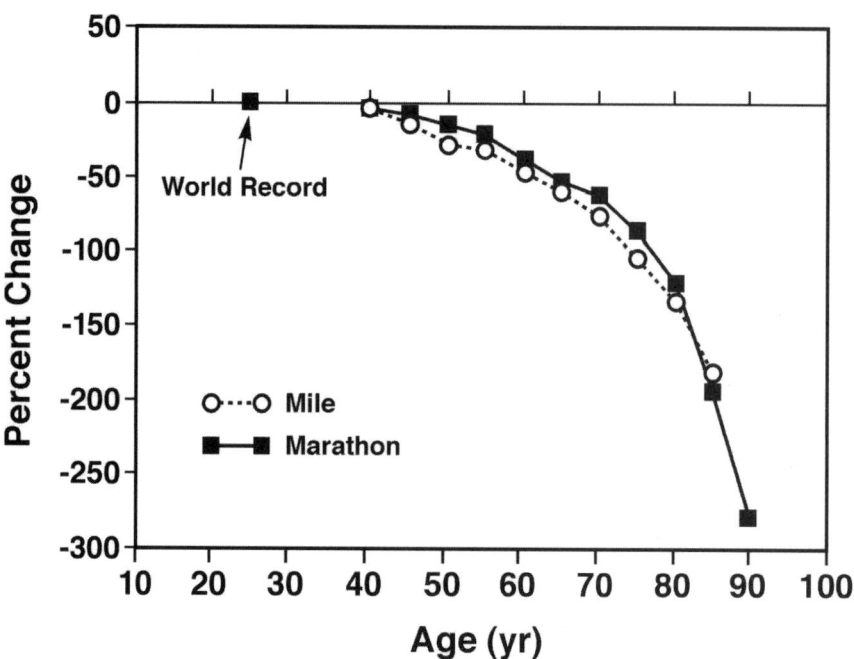

Figure 6-2. Women's decline in performance in the 100 meters and the marathon with age. As with the men, there is a rapid decline in performance after age 70 years. These data show that the rate of decline in running times for sprint and endurance events are almost identical for men and women.

accelerated decline in performance independent of a sprint event (100 meters) or endurance event (marathon). In one decade, from age 70 to 80, the time to run a mile is increased by 2min:44s. These records also show that the decline in performance with age is similar among men and women.

OUR AGING BODIES

Information on runners and/or athletes who have exercised the majority of their lives is limited. The following describes physical traits and how they change with age. The data will be primarily drawn upon from a longitudinal study we recently completed in our laboratory. In the late 1960s and early 1970s several world and national caliber, and recreational distance runners were tested in the Human Performance Laboratory. The main goal at that time was to determine what physical qualities made distance runners successful. Twenty-five years later, we re-examined 54 of these same runners. As one might expect, several changes in lifestyle and body type had occurred over the years. Of great interest to us were the runners who had continued to train and compete for more than 20 years. We also found that some of the runners from the 1960s used running as a recreational tool over the years, while others quit the sport of running for a variety of reasons. These runners and non-runners provide a starting point for understanding changes that occur with our bodies as we age.

Body Composition: A Matter of Size?

Probably one of the most difficult challenges runners face as they age is maintaining a reasonable body weight. While the formula for a healthy body weight is simple; burn as many calories as you eat. Adhering to this doctrine is often times difficult. Body weight is particularly important in the sport of distance running. The most successful runners are very thin with low body weight (as discussed in Chapter 1). Perhaps too thin and light for the majority of runners. The advantage is that less body weight means that less energy will be needed to overcome gravity during running. However, as discussed earlier in this book, attempting to lose too much body weight and neglecting nutritional needs could lead to poorer performances.

While body weight is relevant for distance running, it is only part of the picture. The amount of muscle and fat an individual has is also critical. These components of muscle and fat are often referred to as body composition. Typically, the fat to muscle ratio increases slightly as we age, even in the most dedicated and consistent runners (Figure 6-3).

Initially, these body composition measurements were taken when all these individuals were training for marathons. Twenty-five years later, there was a variety of run training, with some not training at all.

In general it appears that some level of running is beneficial for body weight control with age. Runners who continue to train and compete at a high level can expect a small increase in body weight. The highly trained competitive men we tested had increased their body weight 4 pounds in 25 years. This clearly illus-

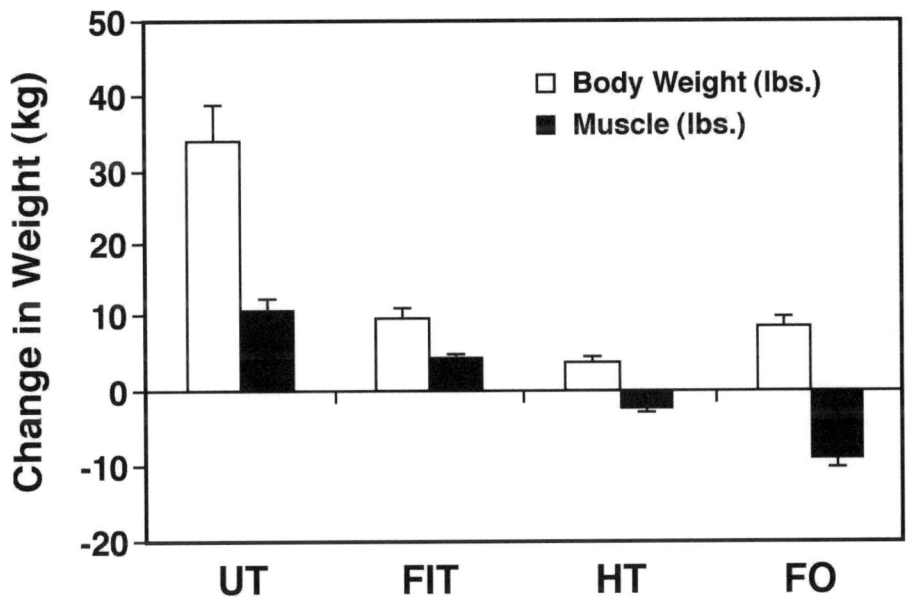

Figure 6-3. Change in body weight and muscle mass over 25 years. All of these men were highly trained when initially tested in the late 1960s and early 1970s. UT = Untrained; FIT = Fitness Trained; HT = Highly Trained; FO = Fit Older Men.

trates that continued distance running is effective for maintaining body size with age. Recreational running also appears to help control body size as we age. The fitness runners had an increase in body weight of 10 pounds in 25 years. Granted, this modest increase in body weight is more than the competitive runners, but illustrates that running for fitness is an effective form of exercise to help minimize weight gain with age.

Not running, however, does little to help control body weight and body fatness. Former marathon runners that had not done any formal training in 10 to 15 years had gained 30 pounds in 25 years. The large increase in body weight was accompanied with an increase in both fat and muscle. The increase in muscle by these non-runners is most likely the result of the extra body weight they had gained. The extra weight they had to carry around each day provided a stimulus for more muscle to be able to handle moving the increased body weight around. While these men were middle-aged when tested, the increased body weight and fat may lead to problems later in life. In fact, the most common type of diabetes is type II (or late onset adult diabetes) that typically results from an inactive lifestyle and too much body fat. Though these men do not exhibit any metabolic complications now, they are targets for future complications, which most likely could be avoided with moderate exercise and reasonable dietary habits.

We were also able to re-test some older runners who were still active in competition. These older men were around 70 years old and had continued to run the majority of their adult lives. These fit older men (as we call them) had a modest change (+9 pounds) in their body weight in 25 years. However, these same older runners also had a decrease in muscle weight of 9 pounds. This suggests that older runners may experience a rather large increase in fat content with an equal loss in muscle content. The reason for this is unclear, but evidence points to changes that occur with protein metabolism with aging. As people get older their metabolism slows down. Part of that slow down process involves a decrease in the making of new muscle proteins. This is a slow process and as a result, people gradually loose muscle mass over time. Why does this happen? We are not sure, but it is related to physical activity, nutrition, and genetics.

Studies have shown that sedentary men and women have a difficult time retaining their muscle mass as they grow older. In contrast, research has shown that men and women more than 90 years old can respond positively to exercise (i.e. resistance training), and increase the size of their muscles. Thus, an apparent paradox exists, that is the older runner that continues to run regularly, but still looses muscle mass. The running should provide enough of a stimulus to promote the making of new muscle proteins for retaining muscle size. However, we have found that older adults do not always eat enough calories to match their energy expenditure. As low-caloric intake habits develop, along with an exercise program, such as running, muscle wasting can result. This phenomenon has been shown in younger adults who are exercising very hard and not eating a good quality diet. The bottom line is that running does not promote increasing muscle size at any age, and as we get older the running may not be a sufficient stimulus to maintain the amount of muscle that we have.

The good news is that middle-aged men and women will benefit from recreational and high level running to help control modifications in body composition with age. However, this does not appear hold true for older (>60 yr) individuals who engage in distance running. Research has shown that older men and women are in jeopardy of losing some of the valuable muscle that they have, even if they continue to run. This is a problem that needs to be addressed in this population.

Cardiovascular Fitness with Aging

As we discussed in Chapter 1, the majority of running occurs at submaximal speeds, but these submaximal efforts are directly influenced by the maximal capacity of the cardiovascular system. This section will discuss how the cardiovascular system is altered during maximal and submaximal running with aging.

Alterations in Cardiovascular Capacity with Aging

1. Aerobic Capacity ($\dot{V}O_2max$)

One of the unique aspects of our 20–25 year follow-up study was that it offered a chance to look at the long-term changes in human physiology in a group of distance runners who have engaged in varied levels of running (or no running at all) over more than two decades. Cardiovascular data from these runners and non-runners showed that everyone could expect a decrease in the maximal oxygen uptake ($\dot{V}O_2max$) with age, regardless of physical activity. However, the decline in $\dot{V}O_2max$ is directly related to the amount and intensity of running performed over the years. Our data from these runners are similar to other cross-sectional studies comparing younger and older runners.

We found the decline in $\dot{V}O_2max$ to vary from as low as 2% in a few runners who had remained fairly consistent with their training and competition to 45% in some individuals who had quit running. Figure 6-4 illustrates the average changes in $\dot{V}O_2max$ for runners and non-runners.

In Figure 6-4, the change in $\dot{V}O_2max$ is represented two ways: 1) ml/kg/min, which is milliliters of oxygen used per kilogram of body weight. This takes into account the runners weight and is probably the best way to represent $\dot{V}O_2max$ since runners have to support and carry their body weight during exercise, and 2) l/min, which is liters of oxygen used per minute. This does not take into account a runner's weight, but is a good way just to look at cardiovascular capacity while running, independent of body weight. So, both ways of expressing $\dot{V}O_2max$ are informative and provide different types of good information about a runner's cardiovascular capacity.

Runners who continue intensive training and competition have a rather small decline in aerobic capacity. Master-level runners that trained hard for

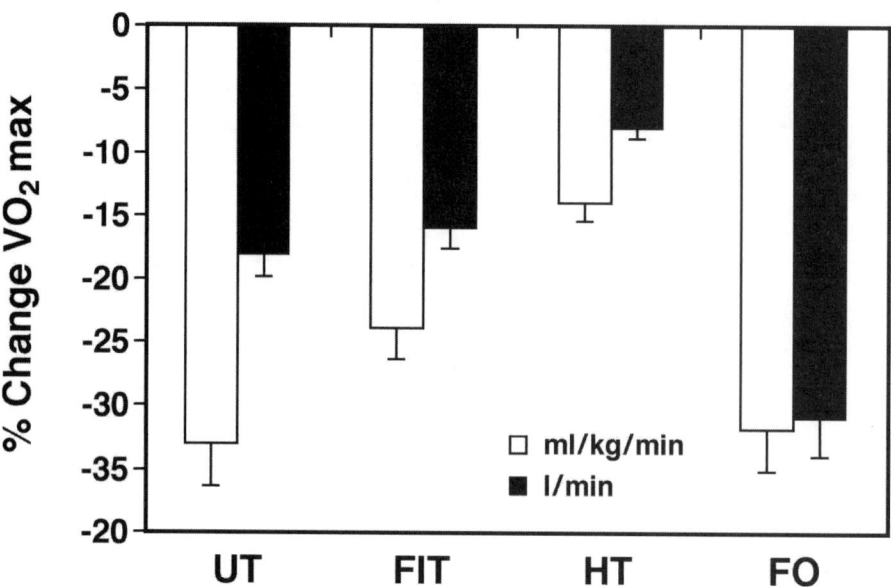

Figure 6-4. Change in maximal oxygen consumption (V̇O₂max) over 25-years in men with varying activity levels. All of these men were highly trained when initially tested in the late 1960s and early 1970s. V̇O₂max is represented in ml/kg/min (corrected for body weight) and l/min (this shows the maximal amount of oxygen that was consumed independent of body weight). UT = Untrained; FIT = Fitness Trained; HT = Highly Trained; FO = Fit Older Men.

most of their adult lives had a 12% reduction in $\dot{V}O_2$max in 25 years. Half of this reduction in $\dot{V}O_2$max was related to the increase in body weight. When the influence of body weight was removed, the drop in $\dot{V}O_2$max was 7%. Since a high $\dot{V}O_2$max has been shown to be one of the critical physiological components of successful distance running, it appears that years of persistent, good quality running are beneficial for a well-conditioned and fairly well maintained cardiovascular system.

Not all the master runners who were training intensely experienced a 12% drop in aerobic capacity. In fact, one of the runners we tested scored a $\dot{V}O_2$max value that was within 2% of his $\dot{V}O_2$max when he was competing and winning marathons (see Side Bar). Derek Clayton, who ran a marathon best of 2h:08min in 1968, was initially tested in 1971 and was found to have a similar cardiovascular profile during his re-testing in 1994. While his training had changed considerably due to orthopedic problems, he still maintained a daily ritual of running intensely 3 to 4 miles a day. This illustrates that years of intense training may be beneficial for maintaining aerobic capacity. These data also confirm previous data in young runners that $\dot{V}O_2$max can be achieved in about 8 weeks and that additional mileage does little to improve $\dot{V}O_2$max (see Chapter 1).

Recreational runners can expect to have a greater decline in aerobic capacity compared to competitive master runners. Fifty-year old recreational runners were found to have a 22% decline in $\dot{V}O_2$max compared to when they were 25 years old. When their $\dot{V}O_2$max was adjusted for the 10 pound increase in body weight, the average decline in aerobic capacity was still 16%. Comparing these data to highly trained runners clearly illustrates that running volume, intensity

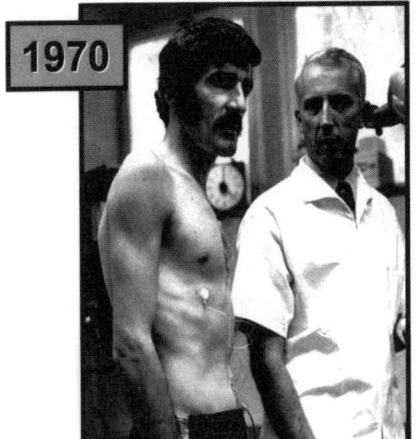

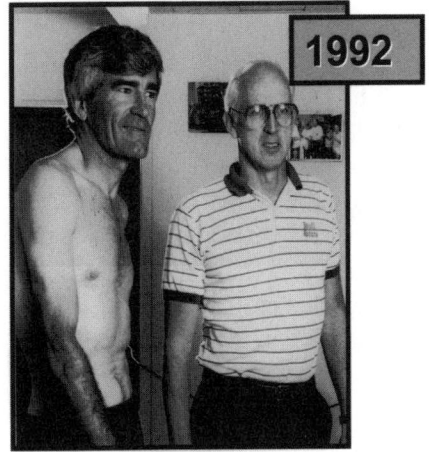

Age = 28 yr
Wt. = 73.1 kg
Fat = 7.1%
$\dot{V}O_2max = 5.09$ l/min
$HR_{max} = 188$ b/min

Age = 50 yr
Wt. = 75.2 kg
Fat = 11.0%
$\dot{V}O_2max = 5.13$ l/min
$HR_{max} = 176$ b/min

and body weight are key components to minimizing a decline in the cardiovascular capacity with aging.

For a number of individuals, lifestyle changes play a key role in their exercise and running habits. We were curious whether former highly trained runners would retain any of their aerobic conditioning when they were older. We tested former marathon runners who had not run for at least 10–15 years and found they had a drop in $\dot{V}O_2max$ of more than 30%. Even though these former runners gained a lot weight over the 25 years, their body weight adjusted $\dot{V}O_2max$ was still 18% lower compared to when they were younger and running marathons. One thing that we noticed was how much these men struggled on the treadmill, not even coming close to the speed and incline they were able to achieve many years earlier. In fact, a couple of men had to stop the running treadmill test early due to chest pain. This is clear evidence that a change to a sedentary lifestyle is detrimental to running performance, cardiovascular function, body weight and also may be problematic to overall health. Furthermore, individuals who cease running do not appear to retain any cardiovascular benefit from the intense marathon training and competition when they were young.

Some of the runners we tested were, on average, 70 years old and still competing in 10K and marathon races. These men offered us a unique opportunity to compare the long-term changes in their aerobic capacity and performances. The aging literature and data on running records suggest that around age 70 is when one can expect to start experiencing a rapid decline in aerobic capacity, muscle strength, and performance. Our data on 70 year old men help to confirm that a large drop-off in physiological capacity occurs even though they had been running their entire adult lives. We found the fit older marathon runners had a 30% decline in $\dot{V}O_2$max despite continuing to train and compete over the 20 to 25 year period. The question is why these men had such a large decrease in their aerobic capacity with continued run training and competition? A possible explanation is the decrease in muscle mass that these men experienced. As noted earlier, these men had lost about 9 pounds of muscle over the 20 to 25 years. With less muscle there is less active tissue during running. Less active muscle tissue also means less active tissue to take up and utilize oxygen during exercise. Thus, it seems reasonable to conclude that part of the drop off in $\dot{V}O_2$max with older runners is related to the loss of muscle tissue that occurs with aging.

Figure 6-5 summarizes the changes in $\dot{V}O_2$max in runners with different training regimens (highly trained, recreational trained, and untrained) and older runners. For comparison purposes, the typical decline in $\dot{V}O_2$max among athletic and sedentary individuals is shown.

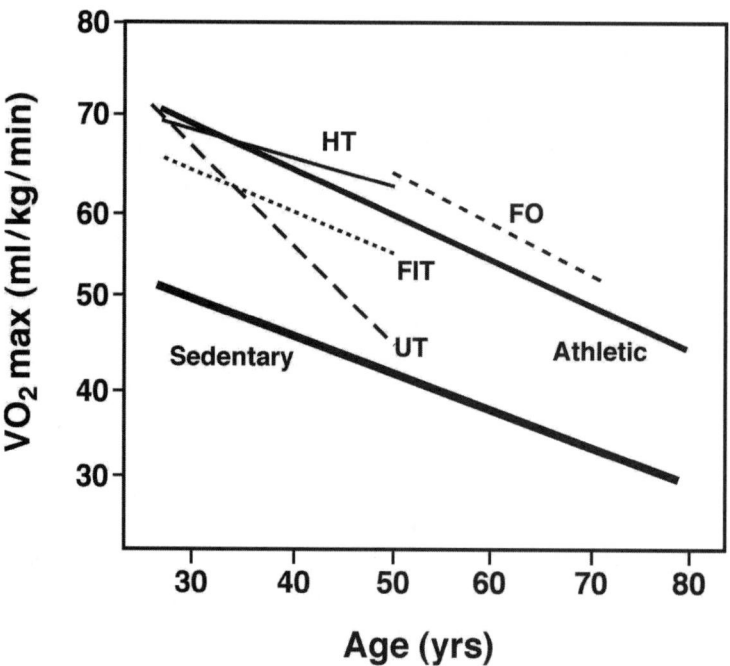

Figure 6-5. *Rate of decline in maximal oxygen consumption (VO₂max) over 25 years in men with varying activity levels. All of these men were highly trained when initially tested in the late 1960s and early 1970s. UT = Untrained; FIT = Fitness Trained; HT = Highly Trained; FO = Fit Older Men.*

2. Maximal Heart Rate and Ventilation

As with $\dot{V}O_2$max, maximal heart rate and maximal ventilation (breathing) is usually lower in all types of runners with age. Vital capacity, another measure of lung volume, is also lower in runners and non-runners and helps explain why maximal ventilation decreases with age. That is, a smaller lung volume (vital capacity) leads to less air that can move through the lungs in a given amount of time (ventilation). In Table 6-3 changes that occur in heart rate, ventilation and vital capacity are shown for runners of different fitness levels.

It is well known that your maximal heart rate will get lower as you age. At the age of 20 years, you might be able to elevate your heart rate to 200 beats/minute during an exhaustive mile or two-mile run. But, by the time you are 50 years old, your maximal heart rate may be down to 170 to 180 beats/minute. In support of this, the 50 year old veteran runners had a maximal heart rate ranging from 174 to 180 beats per minute, independent of fitness level. Older runners (70 year olds) had an average maximal heart rate of 155 beats per minute, which was down from the 175 beats per minute value recorded in the late 1960s. Thus, it appears that fitness level has little control over maximal heart rate with age and other genetic factors playing a more significant role in determining one's maximal heart rate.

Research and anecdotal information show that pulmonary function is reduced in older runners. Why does lung volume decline, as we get older? There is no clear scientific answer to explain the decrease in lung capacity with age. One possibility is that the muscles aiding lung movements are not as strong as they were several years earlier. This may be related to a decrease in the function of those muscles that is caused by aging, or perhaps less intense workouts are not as effective for expanding and contracting the lungs. Another possibility is that the capacity of the lungs has declined due to pollutants inhaled over the years. While the runners we tested were not smokers, they still inhaled a small amount of contaminants over the years that may have slowly affected the lung tissue. The bottom line is that pulmonary function and therefore the capacity to move air in and out of the lungs is gradually reduced, as we get older.

TABLE 6-3. Changes in maximal heart rate, ventilation, and vital capacity over a 25 year period in the same men.

Group	Heart Rate (beats/min)			Ventilation (liters/min)			Vital Capacity (liters)		
	T1	T2	%Δ	T1	T2	%Δ	T1	T2	%Δ
HT	191	180	–6%	151	121	–20%	5.5	4.9	–11%
FT	186	174	–7%	130	109	–16%	5.1	4.2	–18%
UT	187	178	–5%	136	111	–18%	5.0	4.0	–20%
FO	175	155	–11%	125	88	–30%	4.6	3.7	–20%

HT = Highly Trained; FT = Fitness Trained; UT = Untrained; FO = Fit Older Men

Despite a continued level of running and competition, even the most dedicated and gifted runners can expect to have a decline in $\dot{V}O_2$max and pulmonary function. However, the decline in $\dot{V}O_2$max is related to the volume and intensity of running performed. Years of distance running does not appear to alter the age-related decline in lung function and heart rate. Information from master athletes engaged in a variety of running regimens provide insight that continued running at any level is good for the cardiovascular system with the more dedicated runners showing the least decline in $\dot{V}O_2$max.

Running Economy in Master Runners

Running economy is one of the key tools for assessing fitness and talent while running. As discussed in Chapter 1, running economy tells us how much energy is being used to run at slower speeds. The more talented runners consume less oxygen while running at submaximal paces. Historically, an 8min/mile pace has been the most common treadmill speed used in the laboratory to assess running economy. Studies of elite distance runners show that the best runners consume 35 to 39 ml/kg/min of oxygen while running an 8min/mile, which is 45 to 50% of their $\dot{V}O_2$max. Conversely, inefficient runners will consume more than 40 ml/kg/min, with the most inefficient runners ("the plodders") consuming more than 45 ml/kg/min. For these less talented runners, this submaximal running can be as high as 70 to 75% of their $\dot{V}O_2$max. The less economical runners are handicapped by poorer biomechanics and a lower $\dot{V}O_2$max, which helps explain why these runners are using such a large portion of their aerobic capacity.

Does economy of running change as we age? One might expect that oxygen consumption, breathing, and heart rate during a slow-paced run would be slightly greater as you age due to variations in fitness and possible changes in biomechanics. Even the most talented runners modify their training habits as they age and might expect that the cost of running an 8min/mile to be greater. Information obtained from treadmill tests in our laboratory show that running economy is similar in older runners, provided the runners are fit. Older, less fit runners and non-runners use more aerobic energy during submaximal runs.

Highly trained master runners can expect to be as economical at running during submaximal speeds as when they were younger provided they have not had any injuries that have dramatically altered their form (biomechanics). We found competitive master runners consumed 38 ml/kg/min of oxygen with a heart rate of 137 beats per minute while running an 8min/mile on the treadmill. These values were nearly identical to the 38 ml/kg/min and 136 beats per minute from the same paced run on the treadmill 25 years earlier. While these data clearly show that the energy to run an 8min/mile is unchanged with age, the stress to perform this run is greater. Remember that all runners will experience a drop $\dot{V}O_2$max with age. Thus, relative to $\dot{V}O_2$max, the submaximal 8min/mile pace is more stressful. When these runners were 25 years old, they were working at 59% of their $\dot{V}O_2$max during the 8min/mile pace compared to 71% when they were 50 years old. While economy of running does not appear to change in middle-aged master runners the level of stress to perform slower-paced running is greater due to the reduction in aerobic capacity.

Mother nature is not as kind to those who run for fitness or not at all. Since running economy is largely influenced by body weight, middle-aged recreational runners and non-runners are at a distinct disadvantage during submaximal running. The interesting aspect for the master level recreational runners is that they have a similar oxygen uptake and heart rate during an 8min/mile pace compared to highly trained competitive runners. On the surface it would appear that middle-aged recreational runners and highly trained runners have comparable efficiency while running long distances. Upon closer examination, the recreational runner suffers from a greater body weight and lower $\dot{V}O_2$max compared to the more competitive-type master runner. When these factors are taken into account, it becomes obvious that running is much more taxing for the casual runner. To run at an 8min/mile pace, the older fitness runner has to work at nearly 80% of their aerobic capacity. This level of effort is substantially greater than the elite level master runner.

An interesting component older runners possess, is the noticeable running skill that was developed compiling hundreds of miles when they were younger. Even in the most unfit former runners that we have tested, it was obvious that these individuals possessed an inherent talent for running. While these runners were chubby and out-of-shape, you could tell by watching them run on the treadmill that they had a gift for running. This was further reflected in the data from the submaximal 8min/mile treadmill run. Like the highly trained and fitness trained master runners, the former marathon runners had an oxygen cost that was comparable to perform this run. These untrained runners had an oxygen uptake of 42 ml/kg/min while running an 8min/mile. However, most of these untrained runners had a heart rate around 150 beats per minute, which is substantially greater than more fit runners of similar age. As you might expect, when the oxygen cost of an 8min/mile is compared to their $\dot{V}O_2$max value, it becomes clear that running an 8min/mile is barely tolerable. In fact, the untrained former runners were working at 90% of their $\dot{V}O_2$max during the submaximal treadmill run. In other words, they were nearly at maximal effort just to perform an 8min/mile run.

Changes in running economy with age appear to be primarily dependent upon fitness level. While the energy it takes to perform longer runs at a given pace may not change a great deal with age, the stress to perform these runs will increase substantially for all runners. As we get older, the tolerance for holding a descent running pace is determined by changes in $\dot{V}O_2$max and body weight.

SKELETAL MUSCLE FUNCTION WITH AGING

Distance running requires a coordinated effort of several muscles to run. With training, these skeletal muscles are conditioned for the strength and speed requirements for peak running performance. And it is this peak performance that most older runners are attempting to hold on to. The most typical complaint of the master athlete is that they lose their speed, or easy speed. What causes the speed component of running to suffer with aging? Why does the sprinting ability of runners seem to be one of the first traits to be lost as our bodies mature into middle age and beyond? Is the endurance potential of older muscle different? Is there anything that can be done to maintain muscle performance as we age? These are but a few of the questions often asked by veteran runners. This section will focus on what we know about muscle (and don't know) and how muscle responds to training as we age.

Changes in the Runner's Muscle With Age

Probably one of the most notable features associated with aging is the decline in muscle strength. Muscle strength is fairly well maintained until about age 50. Beyond age 50, a steady gradual reduction in muscle function is found. This reduction in strength can limit running performance. Why do we have a reduction in muscle strength? There are several physiological factors that contribute to this decline in muscle performance, but the most obvious culprit is the loss in muscle mass that accompanies the aging process. Several good studies have shown that the total number of muscle fibers in the muscle is reduced in older adults (Figure 6-6).

In younger adults, the thigh muscles have approximately 700,000 individual muscle fibers. After age 50, the number of muscle fibers begins to decline and can be as low as 300,000 in people over 80 years old. That is less than half of the total number of muscle fibers in older adults compared to younger adults! When muscle strength is corrected for muscle size (called specific tension), the normalized strength values are comparable among young and old adults. Thus, it would be a safe assumption that the amount of muscle you have plays an important role in muscle function with age.

As noted earlier, the fit older (70 years of age) runners we studied lost about 9 pounds of muscle mass, indicating that the initial signs of muscle loss were present. We also found these men to have weaker calf muscles. The combination of less muscle mass and strength were part of the reason these older men are not able to perform as well. When you couple the decline in cardiovascular function with the decline in muscle mass and strength of these men, all the ingredients are there to help explain why older people (>60 yrs old) begin to suffer with slower running performances. Does this mean all people over 60 are going to perform poorly? Simply put, no. At least the aging process can be cheated a bit

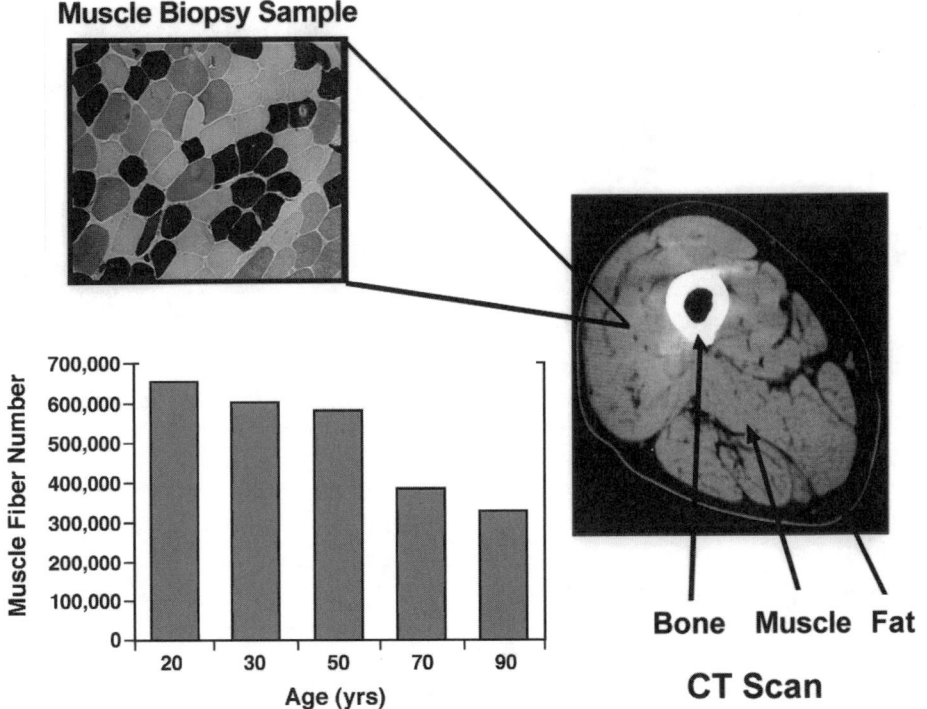

Muscle Biopsy Sample

Bone　Muscle　Fat

CT Scan

Figure 6-6. The bar graph illustrates the impact of aging on the total number of muscle fibers in the thigh muscle of the leg. Shown is a cross-sectional picture of the thigh (CT Scan), and cross-section of muscle fibers from a muscle biopsy sample. Note, that the total number of fibers in the leg is well-maintained until around 50 years of age.

with good dietary habits, continued running, and a moderate lifting program as described later in this chapter. Good genes help too!

It is visually clear from the cross-sectional scans (CT Scans) in Figure 6-7 that the muscle size of the calf among runners with various running mileage, have noticeable differences in their fat distribution surrounding the muscles. When comparing these runners, the recreational and untrained men had more fat surrounding their muscles. This data illustrates that one of the benefits of running is that it helps limit the amount of fat surrounding the leg muscles. Although, as the distance runner ages beyond 60 years old, there is less muscle and more fat. Can this be attributed solely to aging? Most likely, the less muscle and more fat in the runners over 60 years old and beyond is a combination of aging and a decrease in run training.

Research on older runners indicates that continued distance running after age 60 is insufficient to maintain muscle strength and size. Thus, while distance running may be a very good activity for fitness, it is not enough to preserve muscle mass as we get older. That is why some type of regular strength training program would be a wise activity to perform for older runners.

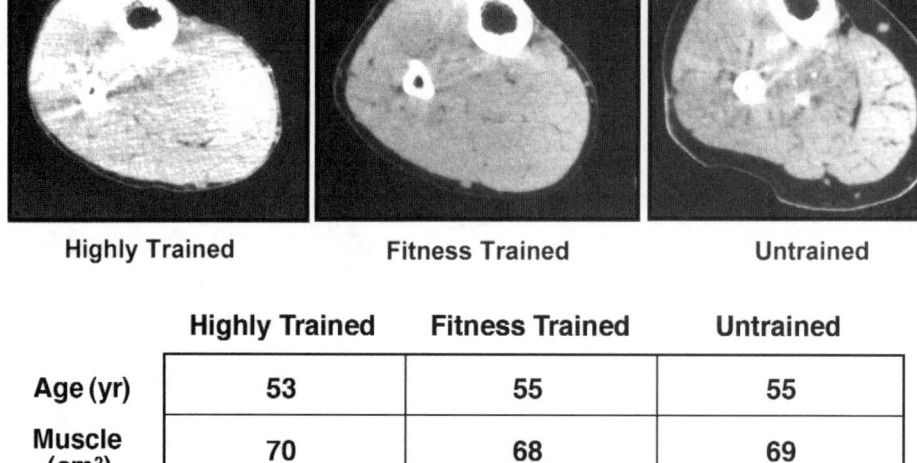

Highly Trained   **Fitness Trained**   **Untrained**

	Highly Trained	Fitness Trained	Untrained
Age (yr)	53	55	55
Muscle (cm²)	70	68	69
Fat (cm²)	8	14	29

Figure 6-7. Three CAT Scan images from the calf muscles of three people of the same age with different activity levels. Note that the amount of muscle for each individual is about the same, while the amount of fat increases with decreasing levels of running or no running at all.

What Should Older Runners Do To Maintain Muscle Mass?

This question is not easy to answer. There is one suggestion; however, that may be helpful for the senior runner; lift weights. This may seem a little elementary, but lifting weights is a proven tool in the fight against losing muscle mass with aging (a condition known as sarcopenia). Furthermore, a strength-training program can be fairly simple and very effective at the same time. As stated above, older men and women have the ability to respond to a resistance-training program by increasing both muscle strength and the amount of muscle that they have (i.e. mass). In fact, older people retain the ability to respond to strength training much the same way younger adults do. The difference among the younger and older adults in performing a strength-training program is that the goals are different. Younger adults typically strength train for recreational purposes to see how big and strong they can become. The goal for older adults is much more practical: lift weights to help maintain muscle function and mass for every day living and hopefully cheat father time and run faster.

There is a variety of weight lifting programs and as many or more opinions on what type of strength training is best. Perhaps the best solution is a simple one. We have found that strength training 1 to 2 days per week is effective in maintaining muscle mass in older adults. But, for this to be effective, the intensity of the strength training must be adequate. What is adequate? Research has shown that 70 to 80% of your maximum effort should be the target intensity. The following are some general guidelines outlining a simple resistance-training program that older runners could use:

144   *RUNNING: THE ATHLETE WITHIN*

1. Lift weights 1 to 2 days per week.
2. Lift the larger muscle groups: Legs, hips, back, arms, shoulders.
3. Lift at 70–80% of your one-repetition maximum (1-RM).

How do you Determine your 1-RM so that you can Lift at 70–80%?

1. Warm-up with a light jog or stationary bike ride (5 to 10 minutes).
2. For a given muscle group (i.e., legs) lift a very light weight a few times.
3. Increase the weight to a moderate amount and lift it 2 to 3 times.
4. Set the weight at an amount that will be difficult to lift and attempt to lift it one time. Then rest for 1 minute.
5. If successful, increase the weight slightly and repeat step 4.
6. If unsuccessful, decrease the weight slightly and repeat step 4.
7. Continue to increase the weight and lift it one time until you cannot complete a given weight. This is your 1-RM.
8. From your 1-RM, you can calculate your 70 to 80% effort:
    Example: 1-RM = 100 lbs., then you should lift 70 to 80 lbs. when you train.
9. Keep a log book, so that you can keep track of your 1-RM values for each muscle group.
10. Approximately once per month, repeat the 1-RM test and re-adjust your 70 to 80% effort. This will help ensure that you are training at the proper intensity.

What Should a Runner do for a Strength-Training Workout?

Typically, for each muscle group, complete 2 to 3 sets with 8 to 10 repetitions per set. Be sure to take 1 to 2 minutes between each set. Complete this for each of the large muscle groups. This workout will only take about 30 to 45 minutes to complete. One other thing to keep in mind that is a common mistake among most people who lift weights: keep proper form. This will not allow you to lift as much weight, but it will target the muscles more effectively and help reduce the risk of injury!

So, for a small investment of 1 to 2 days per week at 30 to 45 minutes each session, your muscles stand to benefit a great deal. Granted, you are not going to get big and win any strength contests any time soon. But that is not the goal. This program will help you to preserve the muscle mass you already have.

Muscle Fiber Composition with Aging and Running

Human skeletal muscle is composed of a mixture of different fiber types (see Chapter 1 for a more comprehensive overview). There are two main fiber types in human muscle: 1) slow-twitch fibers, which are best suited for endurance events and help maintain muscle tone and posture, and 2) fast-twitch fibers which are best suited for explosive events and energy production without oxygen (anaerobic). These fiber types come in a variety of shapes and sizes and understanding how they operate can get fairly complex when examining their protein and functional profile. To keep things simple, these fiber types cover a continuum of functionality and size to perform a variety of tasks. For instance, we have fibers that are small and contract slow (typically slow fibers) and fibers that are large and contract fast (typically fast fibers). There are also several combinations of slow and fast fibers in-between to allow for a wide range of performance.

As we get older, we gradually have fewer and fewer muscle fibers. How we lose these muscle fibers is still a bit of a mystery, but we do not lose all fibers at an equal rate. The fast-twitch muscle fibers are the first to be lost. Not all of them, but the fast-twitch fibers are lost at a greater rate than the slow-twitch fibers. It is thought that slower movement and lack of explosive movement as we get older contributes to this preferential loss of fast-twitch fibers. If these fibers are not recruited (activated) for long periods of time, the body thinks they are not needed anymore and the stimulus to maintain these fiber types is lost. Over time, these fast-twitch fibers gradually shrink up and die. Not a good thing to have happen. As we age there are a greater proportion of slow fibers present due to the loss of the fast fibers.

Distance running does not usually involve quick explosive movements. As a result, the fast fibers get used less and less in older runners. While older runners may continue to run, this type of activity remains insufficient to properly activate a large majority of the fast-twitch fibers. So, it seems reasonable to understand why distance running may be inadequate for preserving the fast-twitch fibers and overall muscle mass. That's why a good strength-training program may be necessary for older distance runners to help maintain the integrity of the fast fibers and help to maintain muscle fiber number and size.

In the early 1970s several distance runners had a muscle biopsy from their calf to examine the muscle fiber composition profile of these athletes. The muscle biopsy procedure was conducted again 25 years later to determine if muscle fiber composition had changed in these older runners. One of the unique aspects of this long-term study with master-level distance runners was that we were able to directly examine certain aspects of skeletal muscle function because of the biopsy technique. When these marathon runners were initially tested in the early 1970s 60 to 85% of their calf muscle fiber were composed of slow-twitch muscle fibers. The best runners tested showed that 70 to 80% of their calf muscle was made up of slow-twitch muscle fibers. The runners that maintained a strict training regimen and competition schedule over the 25 years had little change in their fiber-type profile. In contrast, the other runners who ran for fitness or quit running had a 10% increase in the amount of slow-twitch muscle fibers (Figure 6-8).

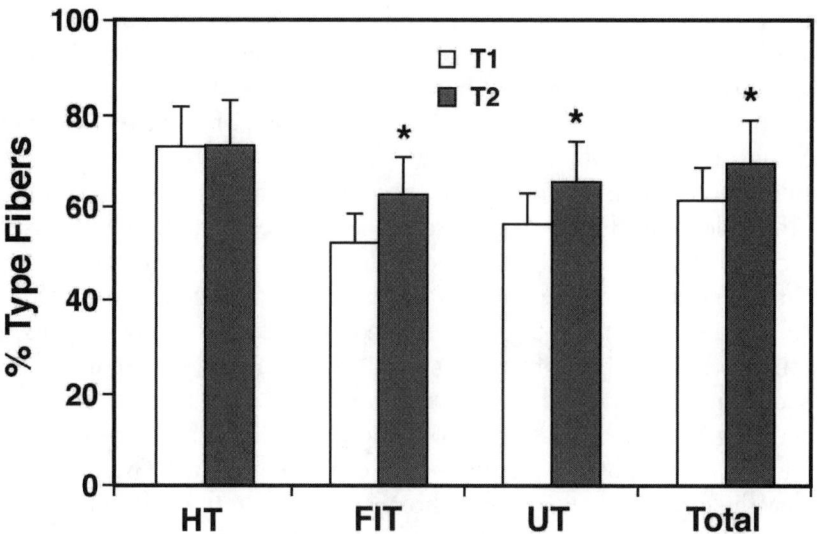

Figure 6-8. *Muscle fiber composition from our original tests (T1 – ~1973) of these men and again 25-years later (T2 – ~1993). The percentage of type I (slow-twitch fibers) is shown. All of these men were highly trained when initially tested in the late 1960s and early 1970s. UT = Untrained; FIT = Fitness Trained; HT = Highly Trained; FO = Fit Older Men. ° Shows a change that was considered significant by scientific standards.*

This data suggests that continued distance running into middle age preserves the muscle fiber type profile of the leg muscles, while decreasing training volume leads to a shift towards more slow-twitch fibers. It is unclear if the shift to more slow-twitch fibers was the result of a fiber transformation from fast muscle fibers to slow muscle fibers, or that at the beginning stages losing fast-twitch fibers occurred, resulting in a relatively greater proportion of slow fibers. At this stage in the life span of these runners (~50 years old), it is difficult to determine if the 10% increase in slow-twitch fibers of the recreational runners and former runners is detrimental for distance running.

Muscle Changes in Elite Distance Runners

In 1974, a distance running camp for the nations best performers was held in Dallas, Texas for training and physiological testing. An extensive skeletal muscle profile was obtained from seven of these elite runners and then repeated again 20 years later. In 1974, these runners were national and Olympic caliber athletes who were training for international competition. Due to their ability, their occupational lifestyles have continued to be related to distance running. All of these men have continued a distance running program at a relatively high volume and intensity over the 20 years. From these men, muscle fiber composition, muscle fiber size, and aerobic potential of the muscle were evaluated. This allowed for a unique examination into how skeletal muscle adapts with training and aging in a group of elite level runners.

Muscle fiber composition for the Dallas runners was compared using the two muscle biopsy samples that were separated by 20 years. In 1974, 81% of their calf muscle was slow-twitch fibers. After 20 years, 76% of their calf muscle was made up of slow-twitch muscle fibers. Thus, the percentage of slow-twitch muscle fibers did not really change in 20 years.

While fiber type did not change in these men, after 20 years of running, the size of their slow-and fast-twitch muscle fibers were smaller. The slow-twitch fibers were 27% smaller, while the fast-twitch fibers were 11% smaller. On the surface, this may appear as a non-desirable trait for running and aging. However, distance running requires a large aerobic component for success in this sport. Part of the oxidative nature of running requires getting the oxygen into the muscle cell and then transported to the mitochondria (a specialized part of the cell for processing oxygen) for energy production. The fact that muscle cells were smaller is probably a positive adaptation for distance running. The smaller fibers mean that the oxygen has to travel a shorter distance in the cell to be useful for making useable energy. This shorter diffusion distance for oxygen may aid in a more efficient muscle cell for aerobic energy production.

The aerobic potential of the muscle for these talented runners was also examined as part of the longitudinal evaluation. A marker of aerobic potential in the muscle cell is an enzyme called succinate dehydrogenase (SDH). We found that the level of SDH in the calf muscle had decreased by about 10% after 20 years. This suggests that oxidative metabolism of the muscle cell may be slightly lower with aging in individuals who continue to endurance train at a relatively high volume and intensity for a 20 year period. However, it should be noted that aerobic enzyme levels in the skeletal muscle from these men were at the upper end of the spectrum for highly trained runners in 1974 and again in 1994. These data indicate that the ability of the skeletal muscle to retain its oxidative potential will remain high if endurance running is continued for a 20 year period.

A New Way To Look At Muscle

Recently, a technique has been developed that allows for a direct examination of contractile function of one muscle fiber. From a muscle biopsy sample, single fibers can be carefully dissected out of a muscle bundle with the aid of a microscope, tweezers, and some steady hands. Once the fiber segment (~3-4 mm long) is removed from the bundle, it is suspended between a motorized arm (this motor can move to manipulate the fiber) and a force transducer (this measures force output of the fiber) and bathed in a relaxing solution in a small chamber (Figure 6-9).

In the relaxing solution, the fiber behaves much the same way it would at rest in the body. At this point the fiber is ready for physiological examination. The fiber is moved into another small chamber that contains a solution with high amounts of calcium (one of the main ions that turns on muscle contraction) and

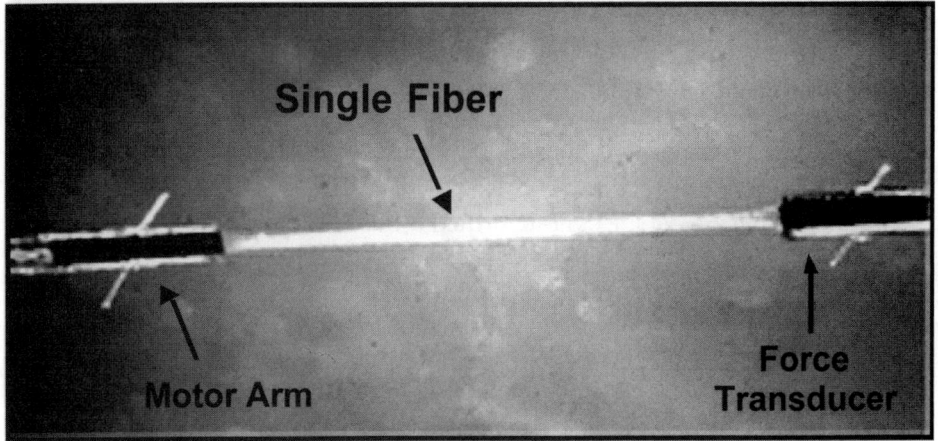

Figure 6-9. A photograph of one muscle fiber suspended between a motorized arm and a force transducer. The muscle fiber segment shown is magnified 400 times normal and is approximately 2 millimeters long.

ATP (the energy currency of the body). A series of contractions and movements of the single fiber allows us to study the contractile properties of that one fiber. From this procedure we can determine the following:

1. How big the muscle fiber is (size).
2. The maximal strength of the fiber.
3. How fast the fiber can contract (contractile velocity).
4. How powerful the fiber is (peak power).

Measuring single fiber function provides us with information that would be similar to the type of information that would be gained from testing whole muscle strength and power components. However, there are several distinct differences and advantages to the single fiber technique.

1. **The nervous system is not involved with these measurements.** This is critical for understanding how muscle behaves with aging and training. As you may recall from earlier in the book, during normal whole muscle contraction, the nervous system sends an impulse to activate a group of muscle fibers. The greater the signal, the more muscle fibers that are recruited and the greater the strength output of the muscle. The single fiber technique eliminates the integration of the muscle and nerve so that the information gained is focused on the operation of the muscle contractile machinery.
2. **Information about the contractile function of individual slow-and fast-twitch muscle fibers can be determined.** In whole muscle measurements, a mixture of slow and fast fibers is stimulated at the same time. As a result, we cannot determine how just the slow muscle fibers or fast muscle fibers are responding. Being able to separate out information

concerning slow-and fast-twitch fiber behavior was important for our understanding of how distance runners' muscle react to a life-time of running and aging.

The single fiber technique is an important physiological advancement for looking at muscle physiology at the cell level. This provides us with detailed information regarding fiber types and contractile behavior without the interference of the nervous system. The only drawback from the technique is the time intensive nature of these measurements. On average it takes two hours to properly study one muscle fiber. In our lab, we attempt to study several fibers from each runner. This adds up to a considerable amount of time and effort. However, the scientific information is novel and it is helping us to better understand runners' muscle and the impact of aging upon muscle function.

Single Fiber Function in Elite Distance Runners

We were fortunate to be able to study single muscle fiber function from the Dallas runners as part of the aging distance runner study. This group represented some of the best masters runners and were all elite level runners when they were younger. For comparison, we examined the single fiber contractile characteristics from age-matched sedentary men. These men had never engaged in regular physical activity. By comparing these two groups, we could estimate the impact of 20 to 30 years of running on muscle function at the cellular level.

On average, the diameter (size) of the slow and fast fibers from the distance runners was 7% smaller compared to the sedentary controls (Figure 6-10). The

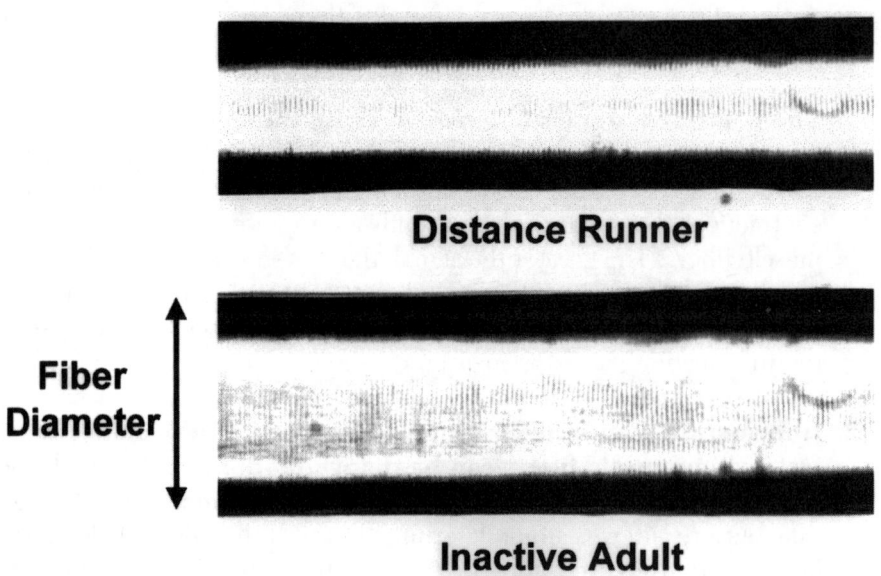

Figure 6-10. Shown is one muscle fiber from a distance runner (~50 years old) and an aged-matched adult who has never engaged in a regular exercise program. The width of the fibers shown is the diameter (size) of each fiber. Note that the distance runner's muscle fiber is smaller compared to the inactive adult. Each muscle fiber shown is magnified 400 times normal.

Distance Runner

Fiber Diameter

Inactive Adult

smaller fibers from the runners were also found to generate less peak force (strength). In fact, the slow and fast fibers were 15% weaker in the runners. However, when the strength of these fibers was corrected for fiber size (specific tension), no differences were observed. Thus, the smaller cell size of the runner's muscle fibers was responsible for the decreased absolute strength.

Contrary to the greater size and strength of the sedentary controls, the contractile velocity of the slow fibers from the runners' fibers was significantly faster. The contractile speed of a single muscle fiber is an indication of how fast a fiber can move or contract. The runner's slow fibers contracted, on average, 19% faster compared to the sedentary men's slow fibers. We did not find any differences in the shortening speed of the fast fibers between the runners and sedentary men. These data indicate that distance running has a greater impact on the physiology of slow fibers. This makes sense, since slow fibers are heavily used during distance running, with little involvement from the fast-twitch muscle fibers.

Power output can also be determined from a single muscle fiber. The measure of fiber power is essentially a combination of the strength and speed components from a given fiber. Despite the elevated contractile speed of the runners' slow fibers, it was still insufficient to overcome the deficits in strength equal to the power characteristics of the sedentary control fibers. The slow and fast fibers from the sedentary controls were 13% and 27% more powerful, respectively, compared to the runners (Figure 6-11).

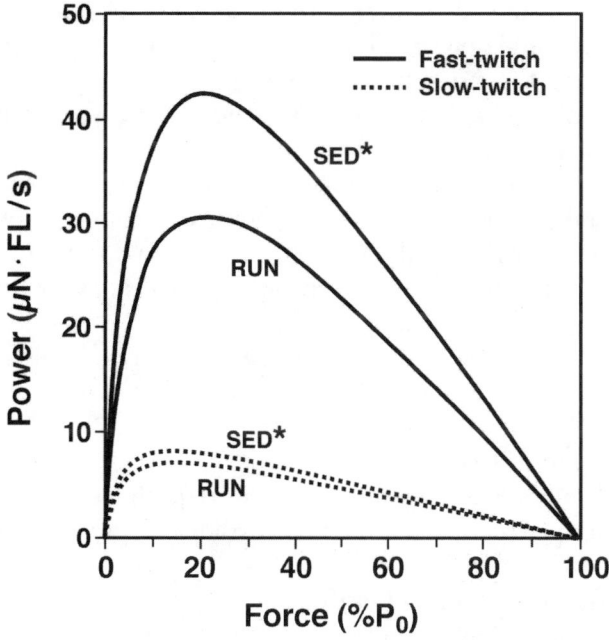

Figure 6-11. Single muscle fiber power of slow-twitch and fast-twitch fibers from distance runners and age-matched adults who have never exercised. Note that the sedentary adults have greater power production from both the slow and the fast fibers compared to the distance runners. Also note the fact that the fast fibers have about a 4-fold greater power output compared to the slow fibers.

From these data it appears that years of distance running causes single muscle fibers to be smaller, weaker, contract faster, and produce less power compared to individuals who lead a normal sedentary lifestyle. While this may seem like a disadvantage for sports performance, it most likely is a physiological adaptation that is advantageous for distance running. The smaller fibers allow for a shorter diffusion distance of oxygen and substrates during exercise. Furthermore, distance running does not require a large strength or power output during exercise, but rather a sustained submaximal power output over a long period of time. Thus, the differences in single cell function among life-long distance runners and sedentary individuals is no doubt an adaptation to years of exercise which have most likely been optimized for the sport of distance running.

ORTHOPEDIC CONSIDERATIONS

In general, running has positive benefits from a fitness and health standpoint, but running posses risks from an orthopedic (joint) perspective. Running places a great deal of stress on the joints involved with absorbing the impact of repeated running strides. In particular, the knee joint and foot are the most susceptible for injuries directly resulting from running. In fact, a number of adults would most likely continue to run if they did not have orthopedic problems. For a lot of people, it gets to the point where running is no longer worth the pain associated with the exercise.

In an attempt to determine the impact of running on joint problems and bone health, we tested all runners and non-runners for degenerative joint disease and bone mineral density. This allowed us to gauge whether running led to negative effects on the musculoskeletal system.

Prevalence of degenerative joint disease was assessed through a medical history and physical examination, injury history, radiologic examination of the knees (graded for joint space narrowing, osteophytes, varus/valgus alignment and subchondral sclerosis), and a comprehensive lower extremity flexibility examination. The following are the highlights found from four different classifications of master runners with an average age of 50, except for the fit older runners who were 70 years old (highly trained (HT), fitness trained (FIT), untrained (UT), and fit older men (FO)) are summarized below:

1. Plantar Fasciitis (PF) — A higher prevalence of PF was noted in the HT (+20%) and FIT (+29%) groups.
2. Medial and/or lateral meniscus injuries requiring surgical intervention — A greater prevalence of this type of orthopedic problem were reported in the FO (57%) and FIT (41%) groups.
3. No differences were identified in hamstring flexibility; however, all groups were below the normal range of 160 to 180 degrees.

4. Radiologic Evaluation — There was a greater amount of osteophyte (bony outgrowth) formation in the 70-year old runners.
5. A greater amount of sclerosis and joint space narrowing were observed in all four groups.

BONE HEALTH

This evaluation involves a scan of the whole body, which provides information about bone strength and density. More specifically, bone mineral density (lumbar and hip regions) using dual energy x-ray absorptiometry (DEXA) was conducted on master runners and non-runners. As can be seen in Figures 6-12 and 6-13, there were no differences in bone mineral density (BMD) or bone mineral

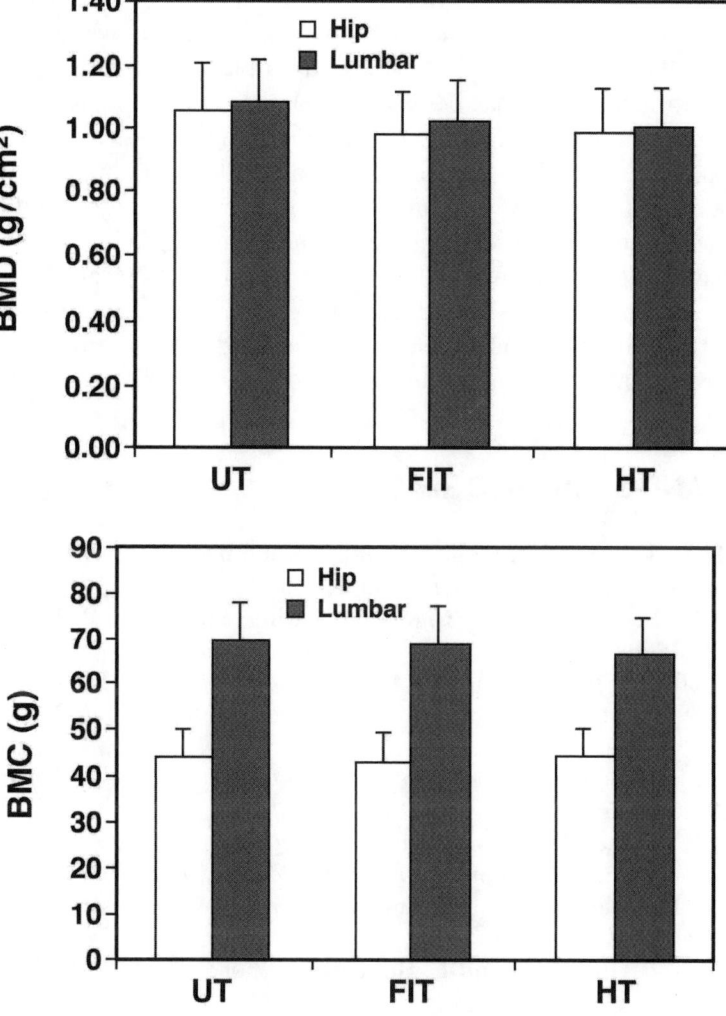

Figure 6-12. Bone mineral density (BMD) of the hip and lumbar (lower back) region of the bones. No differences were found in the density of the bones among these men, suggesting that running does not help or hinder bone density. UT = Untrained; FIT = Fitness Trained; HT = Highly Trained; FO = Fit Older Men.

Figure 6-13. Bone mineral content (BMC) of the hip and lumbar (lower back) region of the bones. No differences were found in the mineral content of the bones among these men, suggesting that running does not help or hinder the mineral content of the bones in middle aged men (~50 y). UT = Untrained; FIT = Fitness Trained; HT = Highly Trained; FO = Fit Older Men.

content (BMC) among the different groups of runners. Interestingly, the bone strength of the runners was no better or no worse than the non-runners. None of the groups had BMD that were different from normative values taken from a general population database. These data indicate that running does not provide any additional advantage for bone strength.

It is apparent that the non-runners in this study were heavier than the distance runners. It has been suggested that heavier men may be protected against osteoporosis. It could be that the greater body mass of the untrained men helped maintain BMD. These data also suggest that distance running does not negatively influence bone density and mineral content.

SUMMARY

The information provided in this chapter has been an overview of some of the changes that occur in the distance runner's physiology with age. From the scientific information that has been gathered, it is rather apparent that continued distance running is beneficial for cardiovascular fitness and muscle function, but may pose a risk to the joints from all of the pounding over the years. For the senior runner (greater than 60 to 70 years old), a more rapid decline in physiological function occurs despite continued running. While the oldest runners we have tested show a marked decline in their physiology and performance, their bodies are much more fit and responsive compared to adults of similar age that do not exercise. So, what should older runners do? Keep running. A lifetime of exercise/running may cheat father time and the aging process a bit!

CLASSIC AND SUGGESTED READINGS

Åstrand I., P-O. Åstrand, I. Hallback and Å. Kilbom. Reduction in maximal oxygen uptake with age. *Journal of Applied Physiology* 35: 649–654, 1973.

Coggan A.R., R.J. Spina, M.A. Rogers, D.S. King, M. Brown, P.M. Nemeth and J.O. Holloszy. Histochemical and enzymatic characteristics of skeletal muscle in master athletes. *Journal of Applied Physiology* 68: 1896–1901, 1990.

Cohen J.J. Apoptosis: the physiologic pathway of cell death. *Hospital. Pract.* 28: 35–43, 1993.

Costill D.L. Metabolic responses during distance running. *Journal of Applied Physiology* 28: 251–255, 1970.

Costill D.L. and E. Winrow. Maximal oxygen intake among marathon runners. *Archives of Physical Medicine and Rehabilitation* 51, 1970.

Costill D.L. Physiology of marathon running. *Journal of American Medical Association* 221: 1024–1029, 1972.

Costill D.L., H. Thomason and E. Roberst. Fractional utilization of the aerobic capacity during distance running. *Medicine and Science in Sport and Exercise* 5: 248–252, 1973.

Dill D.B. Fitness of Harvard men after twenty-two years. *Duke University Council on Gerontology*, 1963, p. 225–239.

Dill D.B. Marathoner DeMar: physiological studies. *Journal of the National Cancer Institute* 35: 185–191, 1965.

Dill B.D., S. Robinson and J.C. Ross. A longitudinal study of 16 champion runners. *Journal of Sports Medicine and Physical Fitness* 7: 4–27, 1967.

Fiatarone M.A., E.C. Marks, N.D. Ryan, C.N. Meredith, L.A. Lipsitz and W.J. Evans. High-intensity strength training in nonagenarians: effects on skeletal muscle. *Journal of the American Medical Association* 263: 3029–3034, 1990.

Frontera W.R., C.N. Meredith, K.P. O'Reilly, H.G. Knuttgen and W.J. Evans. Strength conditioning in older men: skeletal muscle hypertrophy and improved function. *Journal of Applied Physiology* 64: 1038–1044, 1988.

Goodpaster B.H., D.L. Costill, S.W. Trappe and G.M. Hughes. The relationship of sustained exercise training and bone mineral density in aging male runners. *Scand J Med Sci Sports* 6: 216–221, 1996.

Heath G.W., J.M. Hagberg, A.A. Ehsani and J.O. Holloszy. A physiological comparison of young and older endurance athletes. *Journal of Applied Physiology* 51: 634–640, 1981.

Klitgaard H., M. Mantoni, S. Schiaffino, S. Ausoni, L. Gorza, C. Laurent-Winter, P. Schnohr and B. Saltin. Function, morphology and protein expression of ageing skeletal muscle: a cross-sectional study of elderly men with different training backgrounds. *Acta Physiologica Scandinavia* 140: 41–54, 1990.

Larsson L., G. Grimby and J. Karlsson. Muscle strength and speed of movement in relation to age and muscle morphology. *Journal of Applied Physiology* 46: 451–456, 1979.

Lexell J., K. Hendriksson-Larsen, B. Winblad and M. Sjostrom. Distribution of different fibre types in human skeletal muscles: effects of aging studies in whole muscle cross section. *Muscle and Nerve* 6: 588–595, 1983.

Moss R. Sarcomere length-tension relations of frog skinned muscle fibers during calcium activation at short lengths. *Journal of Physiology (London)* 292: 177–192, 1979.

Pollock M.L., H.S. Miller and J.H. Wilmore. A profile of a champion distance runner: age 60. *Medicine and Science in Sports* 6: 118–121, 1974.

Pollock M.L., C. Foster, D. Knapp, J.L. Rod and D.H. Schmidt. Effect of age and training on aerobic capacity and body composition of master athletes. *Journal of Applied Physiology* 62: 725–731, 1987.

Robinson S. Experimental studies of physical fitness in relation to age. *Arbeits Physiologie* 10: 251–323, 1938.

Robinson S., D.B. Dill, R.D. Robison, S.P. Tzankoff and J.A. Wagner. Physiological aging of champion runners. *Journal of Applied Physiology* 41: 46–51, 1976.

Rogers M.A., J.M. Hagberg, W.H. Martin, A.A. Ehsani and J.O. Holloszy. Decline in $\dot{V}O_2$max with aging in master athletes and sedentary men. *Journal of Applied Physiology* 68: 2195–2199, 1990.

Saltin B. and G. Grimby. Physiological analysis of middle-aged and old former athletes. *Circulation* XXXVIII: 1104–1115, 1968.

Trappe S.W., D.L. Costill, W.J. Fink and D.R. Pearson. Skeletal muscle characteristics among distance runners: a 20-yr follow-up study. *Journal of Applied Physiology* 78: 823–829, 1995.

Trappe S.W., D.L. Costill, M.D. Vukovich, J. Jones and T. Melham. Aging among elite distance runners: a 22-yr longitudinal study. *Journal of Applied Physiology* 80: 285–290, 1996.

Trappe S.W., D.L. Costill, B.H. Goodpaster and D.R. Pearson. Calf muscle strength in former elite distance runners. *Scand J Med Sci Sports* 6: 205–210, 1996.

Trappe S., D. Williamson, M. Godard, D. Porter, G. Rowden and D. Costill. Effect of resistance training on single muscle fiber contractile properties in older men. *Journal of Applied Physiology* 89: 143–152, 2000.

Trappe S., M. Godard, P. Gallagher, C. Carroll, G. Rowden and D. Porter. Resistance training improves single muscle fiber contractile function in older women. *Am J Physiol Cell Physiol* 281: C398–406, 2001.

Trappe S.W., T.A. Trappe, G.A. Lee and D.L. Costill. Calf muscle strength in humans. *Int J Sports Med* 22: 186–191, 2001.

Widrick J.J., S.W. Trappe, C.A. Blaser, D.L. Costill and R.H. Fitts. Isometric force and maximal shortening velocity of single muscle fibers from elite master runners. *American Journal of Applied Physiology* 271 (Cell Physiol. 40): C666–C675, 1996.

Widrick J.J., S.W. Trappe, D.L. Costill and R.H. Fitts. Force-velocity and force-power properties of single muscle fibers from elite master runners and sedentary men. *American Journal of Applied Physiology* 271 (Cell Physiol. 40): C676–C683, 1996.

Williamson D.L., M.P. Godard, D. Porter, D.L. Costill and S.W. Trappe. Progressive resistance training reduces myosin heavy chain co-expression in single muscle fibers from older men. *Journal of Applied Physiology* 88: 627–633, 2000.

Chapter 7
Optimizing Performance

INTRODUCTION

Endurance training alone does not insure that you will always run the best possible race. To tell you that there is a "perfect formula" that will lead to a good result every time you race would be a real stretch of the truth. In fact, we all have our good days and bad days. Why this happens still eludes our studies of running physiology. Maybe that is because there is more to it than physiology. However, in order to increase the odds of reaching your best, there are a number of things that appear crucial to helping you achieve your full potential. In other words, there are some aspects of training and reduced training that we know are essential for race preparation. Factors such as improper nutrition, overtraining, and poor pacing during a race can negate many of the qualities gained through months of preparation. In this chapter we will discuss factors that must be monitored and properly managed for runners to do their best.

TOO MUCH OF A GOOD THING

Managing one's training regimen requires more than scientific data. Every training plan must take into account the subjective feel for the runner's response to the stress of training. The goal should be to design a training regimen that provides the level of stress needed for optimal physiological improvements without exceeding the runner's tolerance. Although most runners employ a set of intuitive standards to gauge the volume and intensity of each training session, few are able to assess the relative stress level on the athlete. By the time most runners realize that they have overstressed themselves, it is too late. The damage done by repeated days of excessive training can only be repaired by days and, in some cases, weeks of reduced training or complete rest.

It seems that the runners most susceptible to overtraining or staleness are those who are the most highly motivated, attempting to run hard during every training session or racing too often. You must realize that a sudden increase in training mileage or intensity or both may overload the body's normal processes of adaptation.

Historical Note

Prior to 1972 international rules forbid marathon runners from taking any fluids for the first 10 miles of the race. This was in spite of the scientific evidence that dehydration and heat stroke were likely to occur in this period. Fortunately, pressures exerted by sports physiologists forced the international governing bodies to change this ruling. However, in the late 1980s cases of excessive fluid intake were found to cause a dilution of the runner's blood sodium (hyponatremia), resulting in convulsions and the risk of death.

Symptoms of Overtraining

Though the symptoms of excessive training, often termed "overload training" or "overtraining", may vary from one runner to another, the most common are a feeling of heaviness and an inability to perform well during training and racing. Generally, overtraining and overload training exhibit similar symptoms. These symptoms may include one or more of the following: (1) body weight loss with decreased appetite; (2) muscle tenderness; (3) head colds or allergic-like reactions or both; (4) occasional nausea; or (5) elevated resting heart rate or blood pressure or both.

Psychologically, runners who are excessively trained may exhibit symptoms of depression, irritability, and anxiety. The most common complaint among these runners is that they have trouble falling asleep or that they awaken frequently during the night for no apparent reason. Overtraining results in abnormal psychological, physiological, and performance responses.

The underlying causes of overtraining, also called "staleness" are often a combination of emotional and physical factors. Studies in the early 1950s noted that a breakdown in one's tolerance of stress can occur as often from a sudden increase in anxiety as from an increase in physical distress. The emotional demands of competition, the desire to win, fear of failure, unrealistically high goals, and the expectations of coaches and fellow runners can be sources of intolerable emotional stress. Sources of physical stress include, not only exercise and training, but also environmental temperature, altitude, and improper nutrition.

Day-to-day variations in the sensations of fatigue should not be confused with overtraining. It is not uncommon for a runner's legs to feel heavy after several days of hard training or after a stressful race. Unlike the feelings of being stale or overtrained, the short-lived sensations of heaviness are usually relieved with a day or two of easy training and a carbohydrate-rich diet. Overtraining, on the other hand, is accompanied by a loss in competitive desire and a diminished enthusiasm for training.

There are few warning signs of overtraining. Most of the symptoms are subjective and identifiable only after the runners have overextended themselves. We have observed that runners who suddenly begin to perform very well during training may be on the verge of disaster. They feel so good during training that they tend to extend themselves beyond their day-to-day tolerances, resulting in performance breakdowns.

Diagnosing Overtraining

A number of investigators have used various physiological measurements to diagnose overtraining. Unfortunately, none has proven totally effective. It is often difficult to determine whether the measurements are abnormal and related to overtraining or simply the normal physiological responses to repeated days of hard training.

Measurements of blood enzyme (those molecules that help speed the production of energy) levels have been used to diagnose overtraining with only limited success. Such enzymes as CPK (creatine phosphokinase), LDH (lactate dehydrogenase), and SGOT (serum glutamic oxaloacetic transaminase) are important in muscle energy production but are generally confined to the inside of the cells. The presence of these enzymes in blood suggests some damage to or structural change in the muscle membranes. Following periods of heavy training, these enzymes have been reported to increase two to 10 times the normal levels. Recent studies tend to support the idea that these changes in blood enzymes may reflect varied degrees of muscle tissue breakdown. Examination of tissue from the leg muscles of marathon runners has revealed that there is remarkable damage to the muscle fibers after training and marathon competition. The onset and time course of these muscle changes seemed to parallel the degree of muscle soreness experienced by the runners.

The electronmicrograph presented in Figure 7-1 shows a sample of the damage done to some muscle fibers as a result of marathon running. In this case the cell membrane or sarcolemma has been totally ruptured, with its contents floating freely between the other normal fibers. Though not all of the damage done to the muscle cells is as severe as that shown in Figure 7-1, there are other examples of disruptions within the fibers.

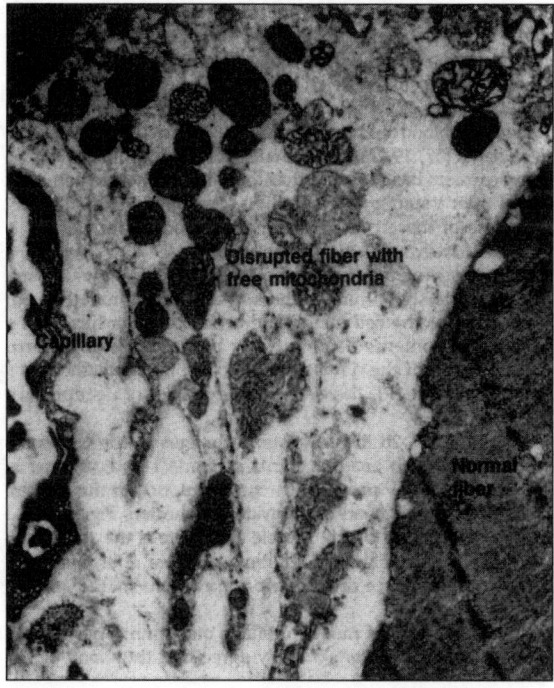

Figure 7-1. An *electronmicrograph of a muscle sample taken immediately after a marathon, showing the disruption of the fiber membrane.*

Figures 7-2a and 7-2b illustrate some changes in the contractile filaments or Z-lines, which are the points of contact and support for the contractile proteins. They provide structural support for the transmission of force when the muscle fibers are activated to shorten. Figure 7-2a shows the normal ultrastructure of the muscle fiber before the marathon race, with the Z-lines intact. Figure 7-2b shows Z-lines after the marathon, pulled apart from the force of eccentric contractions or the stretching of tightened muscle fibers.

Although the effects of running on muscle damage are not fully understood, experts generally agree that microscopic damage to the fibers is common among distance runners. It is also considered to be responsible for localized muscle pain, tenderness, and swelling associated with muscle soreness. There is, however, no evidence that this condition is linked to the symptoms of overtraining. We suspect that blood enzyme levels rise and muscle fibers are frequently damaged during training and competition. Unfortunately, there are no reliable tests that can determine the quantitative damage to muscle or its impact on performance.

Early studies have reported abnormal resting electrocardiographs (EKG) among swimmers who showed signs of overtraining. Typically, those swimmers who showed sudden decrements in performance often exhibited T-wave inversions. Since such EKG changes are associated with abnormal repolarization of

Figure 7-2a. An electronmicrograph showing the normal arrangement of the actonmyosin filaments and Z-line configuration in the muscle of a runner before a marathon.

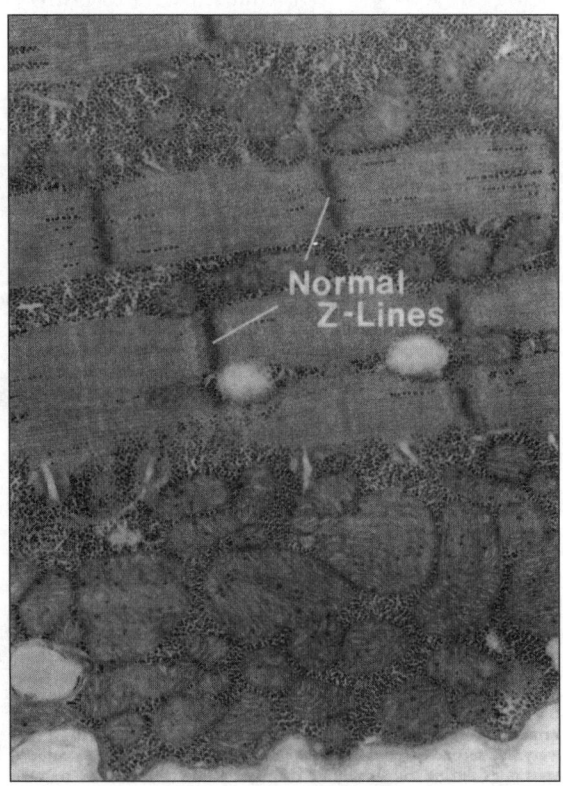

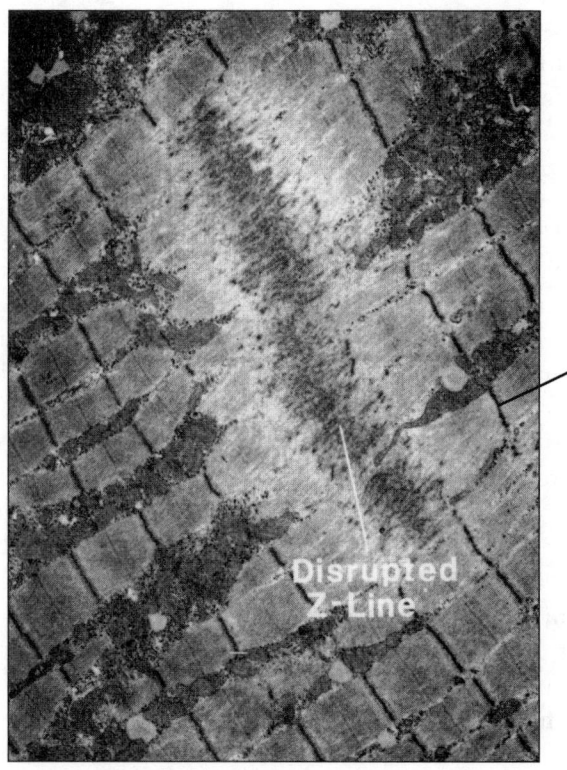

Normal Z-Line

Disrupted Z-Line

Figure 7-2b. An example of Z-line streaming caused by the eccentric contractions of running. This sample of muscle was taken immediately after a marathon race.

the heart ventricles, it was suggested that these changes among training athletes may reveal signs of overtraining. On the other hand, a number of the swimmers who clearly exhibited symptoms of overtraining had normal EKG tracings.

In the mid-1970s we recorded the EKGs of top American distance runners and noted that at least 25% of them had abnormal tracings. These abnormalities, though clinically questionable, appeared to be normal among this highly trained group of male runners. The point here is that what might appear abnormal among untrained, normally active men and women might be common, and inconsequential in highly fit individuals.

Despite various attempts to objectively diagnose overtraining, no single physiological measurement has proven 100% effective. Since performance is the most dramatic indicator of overtraining, we have monitored runners' physiological reactions during a standard, submaximal six-minute mile run. When they show symptoms of overtraining, their heart rates and oxygen consumption during the runs were significantly higher.

One case in particular made this point very clear. Some years ago we observed a college cross-country runner who had an oxygen uptake of 49 ml/kg × min. and heart rate of 142 beats per minute while running a submaximal, six-minute mile. During the same period of this test, his best performance for the 10K was 30min:53s, which ranked him as the third best runner on the team.

Later in the season his 10-kilometer performance deteriorated to 32min:10s, placing him eighth on the team. At that time it cost him significantly more to run the six-minute mile test, 56 ml/kg × min, with a heart rate of 168 beats per minute (Figure 7-3). Interestingly, his maximal oxygen uptake of 70 ml/kg × minute was not changed, despite the diminished performance. While the first six-minute mile required him to work at 70% of his $\dot{V}O_2$max, the same run required 80% of his $\dot{V}O_2$max when he exhibited the symptoms of overtraining. In terms of aerobic fitness, overtrained runners do not lose their conditioning, but they may demonstrate a deterioration in running form. Though the causes for this loss in running skill are not fully understood, overtraining may cause some local muscular fatigue through selective glycogen depletion, forcing runners to alter their mechanics to achieve the same pace.

Although it is impractical for most coaches and runners to consider measuring oxygen uptake during a standardized treadmill run, current technology does make it relatively easy to record heart rate (Figure 7-4). Chest leads pick up the electrical impulses from the heart and transmit them to a recording memory system on the runner's wrist. As the runner performs an evenly paced mile run, the recording system stores heart rates every five seconds. The data presented in Figure 7-5 illustrate a runner's heart rates during the six-minute mile test at the beginning of training, after training, and during a period when he demonstrated symptoms of being overtrained.

Figure 7-3. Oxygen uptake during maximal ($\dot{V}O_2$max) and submaximal (6-min / mile) running during two periods of the season for a college cross-country runner. Note that there was no change in the runner's $\dot{V}O_2$max, despite a markedly slower time for 10 km. At the same time, the amount of energy needed to run at the submaximal pace was notably greater when he appeared to be overtrained.

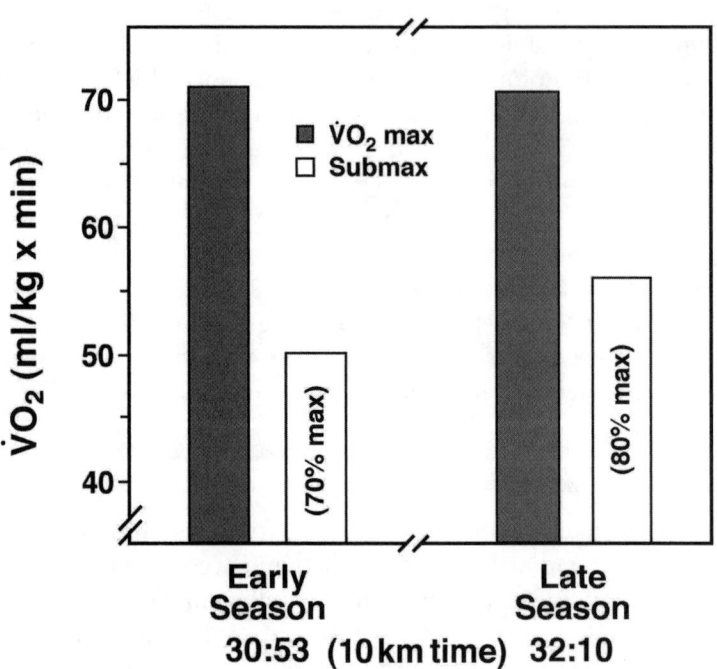

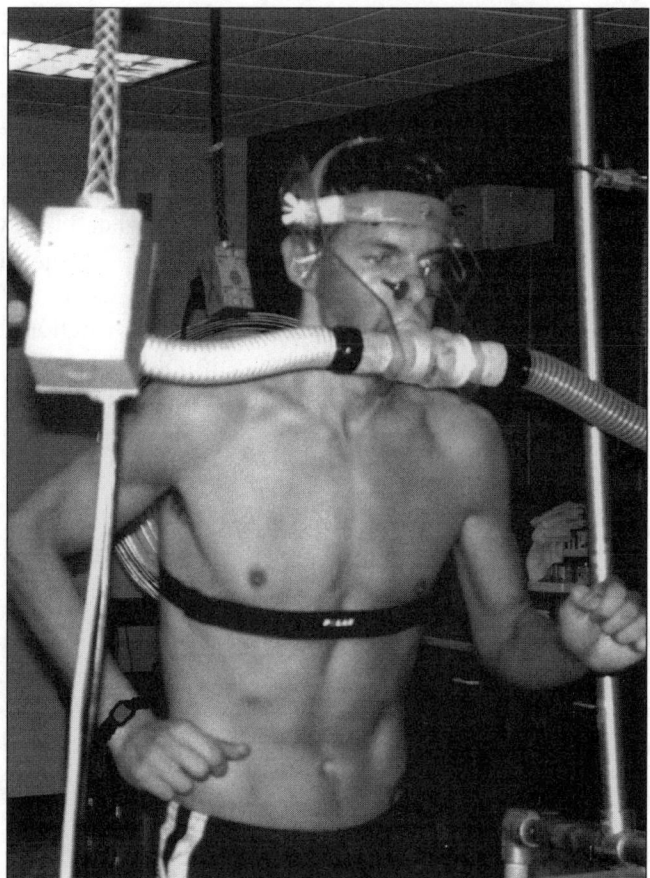

Figure 7-4. *A runner wired to record his heart rate during a standard paced run. The chest strap picks-up and transmits the electrical impulses from his heart to the memory device worn on his wrist. After the run the recording can be replayed for interpretation.*

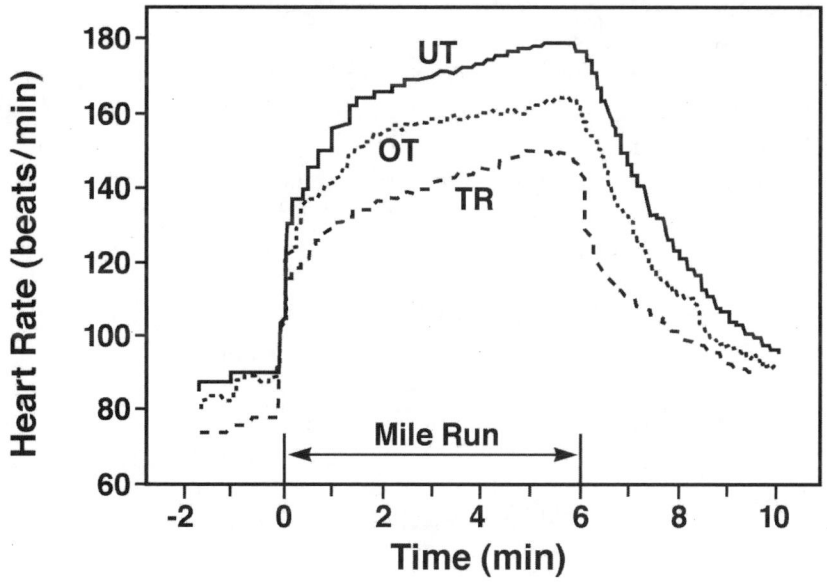

Figure 7-5. *Heart rate responses during a standard, 6-min / mile, submaximal run before training (UT) after a period of training (TR), and during the period when the runner exhibited symptoms of being overtrained (OT).*

Although we use a six-minute mile test with the college runners, a similar test might be performed at eight or nine minutes per mile for less skilled runners. The advantage of this test is that it provides an objective measurement of the runner's physiological response during a set pace. By recording heart rates during and immediately after such a run, it may be possible to objectively determine the runners' fitness for competition. In addition, blood lactate measurements taken after such a test appear to correlate closely with the runner's heart rate. If the runners' heart rate is higher than normal during the standard mile run, we generally find his/her blood lactate is also elevated. Since heart rates are simpler to record and provide immediate information for the runner, it is much more practical to rely on heart rates to monitor any changes in the runner's fitness and may provide a warning signal of overtraining.

MONITORING TRAINING STRESS

Preventing overtraining is a matter of anticipating other stresses and taking care to eliminate them before they take their toll on the runner's performance. What may be stimulating and enjoyable to one runner may add excessive stress to another. This fact makes it nearly impossible to eliminate the problem of overtraining in sports. Only with careful monitoring of the runners' attitudes and performances can we hope to minimize the risk of a breakdown in the system of adaptation. Runners must consider the pace, distance, and accumulated stresses of their training plans. In an effort to objectively evaluate the physical stress imposed by a given workout, we have attempted to generate an equation that can give us an objective index of training stress. Though we admit it is not without its limitations, the following equations can provide an easy evaluation of the demands of a given training session.

First, this program considers the runner's physiological ability ($\dot{V}O_2max$) and his or her current state of training. As mentioned in Chapter 1, $\dot{V}O_2max$ can be predicted from running performance in the mile, two-mile, or 10-kilometer. The relative intensity of the training run can be calculated as the percentage of $\dot{V}O_2max$ used during the run. The oxygen uptake during the training run must be calculated from the equation:

$$\dot{V}O_2 = (329/P) - 5.24$$
where P = running pace in minutes per mile

(example: at 6 minute/mile the $\dot{V}O_2$ = 49.6 ml/kg per minute)
$$\% \dot{V}o_2max = (\dot{V}O_2 / \dot{V}O_2max) \times 100$$

$\dot{V}O_2max$ is calculated as described in Chapter 1.

In order to rate the pace or intensity of a given run, the percent $\dot{V}O_2$max is divided by 70%, a level of effort known to be neither hard nor easy for the runner. If, for example, the runner trained at 70% $\dot{V}O_2$max, then the training intensity (IR) would be rated as 1.0 (70/70 = 1.0). On the other hand, a training pace requiring 85% $\dot{V}O_2$max would be given a rating of 1.21, a more stressful pace.

To rate the distance of a given workout, the mileage is divided by five miles, a distance known to be neither hard nor easy for the runner. If the runner has been averaging five miles per day for the last few weeks, then he or she would be given a distance rating (DR) of 1.0 (5 miles/5 miles) for a five-mile run. If the runner did a training run of seven miles, then the distance rating would jump to 1.40, a marked increase in training stress.

The distance rating and the intensity rating help to estimate the demands of training. Although these two factors may offer different levels of stress, we average the two ratios in an effort to obtain one overall rating (Tl) for the workout. Finally, the overall rating is multiplied by 100 to eliminate decimals.

$$Tl = 100((DR + IR)/2)$$

The advantage of this approach is that it provides a single index of the physiological demands placed on the runner, a rating that can be used to plan subsequent training sessions. Workouts that receive an overall rating above 105 are usually quite stressful, indicating a need for lighter training on the following day. A workout rated at 100 or less is usually tolerated well by runners and can be repeated for several days.

As noted earlier, progressive improvements in conditioning can only be achieved by a systematic increase in mileage and speed. Such an approach, however, necessitates that the training program be closely monitored to ensure this progression and to reduce the risk of overtraining the runner.

Tapering: Reduced Training for Optimal Performance

Though all the causes of overtraining are not clear, it appears that the intensity or speed of training is a more potent stressor than training mileage. As we have pointed-out, relief from overtraining only comes with a marked reduction in training pace or complete rest. Although most coaches suggest a few days of slow, easy training runs, we are inclined to feel that runners recover their running form faster when they rest completely for three to 5 days or engage in some other form of low-intensity exercise like walking. In some cases, counseling may be needed to help the runner cope with job, school, or social pressures, since the runners often experience psychological changes when they are overtrained. At other times the problem may simply be a matter of poor nutrition, insufficient sleep, or both. If the runner shows continued signs of fatigue and substandard performances despite rest and counseling, medical help should be sought.

A leading swimming coach, Ernie Maglischo, has stated that "prevention is always preferable to curing an overtrained state." The best way to minimize the risk of overstressing is to follow cyclic training procedures by alternating easy, moderate, and hard periods of training. Chapter 4 discussed the value and incorporation of rest in the training program. Although there are broad individual variations in the tolerance limits, even the strongest runners have periods when they are susceptible to overtraining. As a rule, one or two days of intense training should be followed by an equal number of easy, aerobic training days. Likewise, a week or two of hard training should be followed by a week of reduced mileage with little or no emphasis on anaerobic running. In addition, special attention should be given to the runner's carbohydrate intake to minimize the risk of chronic muscle glycogen depletion. As noted in Chapter 3, repeated days of hard training will result in a steady decline in muscle glycogen.

Peaking for Performance

Since peak performance requires a sharpening of both physical and psychological tolerance to the stress of running, the runner should be permitted some relief from the chronic demands of training. During periods of frequent competition, most runners take several days of light training and rely on carbohydrate-rich diets to boost their performances. In light of our previous discussions about training, overtraining, and carbohydrate loading, one might question whether these brief periods of tapering are adequate to promote optimal performance. Experience in other sports, such as swimming, suggests that the taper period may need to cover two or more weeks for best results.

Periods of intense training reduce muscular strength, lessening the performance capacity of athletes. To compete at their peak, many athletes reduce their training for five to 21 days before a major competition. Although such a regimen is widely practiced in a variety of sports, most runners fear the loss of conditioning and top running form if they reduced training for such a long period before a major race. A number of studies make it clear, however, that this fear may be unwarranted.

Maximal oxygen uptake can be maintained at the training level with a two-thirds reduction in training frequency. It appears that a greater amount of work is needed to increase $\dot{V}o_2max$ than to maintain it at the trained level. Whereas $\dot{V}o_2max$ and the ability to perform exercise are measurably improved within a few weeks of training, the rate of decline in physical performance with reduced training is much slower.

Swimmers who reduced their training by more than 70% over a 15-day period showed no loss in $\dot{V}o_2max$ or endurance performance. Measurements of blood lactate after a standard 400m swim were actually lower after the taper period than before. More importantly, the swimmers showed an average improvement in performance of 3.5 to 3.7% as a result of the reduced training.

But what does this mean to the distance runner? If a runner were to improve 3.5% after tapering, then a 40-minute 10K runner would be expected to run the same distances in 38min:48s. Unfortunately, studies with runners have not proved to be so predictable. In one of the first studies with runners, three weeks of reduced training resulted in no change in racing times for 5K or $\dot{V}O_2$max, but running time to exhaustion on the treadmill improved 9.5%. However, in a later study, this same investigator found a 3% improvement in 5K time and running economy with just 7 days of tapering. Likewise, studies with 1500-meter runners who tapered for 7 days were able to improve their running time to fatigue by 22%. So, it looks as if tapering works for runners, and may hold promise of better performances. However, research seems to indicate that a 7-day taper may be quite adequate for runners in races of 5K or less. At the present time, there is no information to say whether runners who compete in longer events (i.e., 10K to marathon) will experience the same benefits of tapering.

During our studies with swimmers we noted that the most notable change during the taper period was a significant gain in muscular strength. As a consequence of reduced training, the swimmers demonstrated an increase in arm strength and power of 18 to 25%. Muscle biopsy studies with runners and swimmers have shown that this gain in strength/power after tapering is the result of the individual fibers contracting at higher speeds, thereby producing more power. This change within the leg muscles enable the runners to generate more force and provide them with a feeling of "easy speed."

One characteristic side effect of a prolonged two- or three-week taper is that runners and swimmers experience periods of fatigue and seem unable to extend them during training. Surprisingly, this is the opposite of what we might expect, but it may simply reflect a change in the athletes' psychological state and a subconscious inability to stress themselves. It is interesting to note that on the day of the race, the runners find their usual running pace to be nearly effortless. Their biggest problem seems to be in controlling their pace, since they tend to run too fast in the early stage of the race, thereby resulting in early fatigue in the latter stages of the race.

Table 7-1 offers a two-week tapering plan. Although this taper schedule assumes that the runner has been training an average of eight miles per day, six days per week, a similar plan can be calculated for runners who have been doing more or less by using a similar percentage decrease in the daily training mileage.

During the taper period, keep the fast running to a minimum and eliminate all painful, highly anaerobic workouts. This does not mean that the training excludes all race-pace running. On the contrary, it is important to inject a few paced runs into each workout, but the rest and distance of these runs should be controlled to allow the runner to perform each one without feeling overly tired. The runner should be able to recover quickly from each workout during the taper period. We can not exclude the possibility that part of the improvement in

TABLE 7-1. A sample tapering program in preparation for a 10K race. The runner used in this example had been averaging 8 miles of running per day, six days per week for 6–8 weeks prior to this taper period. The percentage values (%DEC) show the amount of change in training as compared to the runner's average daily mileage.

Day	Mileage	%DEC
Avg. Training	8 miles/day	—
1	5 mile (Ae); 4 × 800 m/2 min rest	–12%
2	4 mile (Ae); 4 × 400 m/1 min rest	–38%
3	5 mile (Ae)	–38%
4	4 mile (Ae)	–50%
5	3 mile (Ae); 2 × 1 mile/4 min rest	–38%
6	REST (No Running)	
7	2 mile (Ae); 3 × 1.5 mile/5 min rest	–19%
8	4 mile (Ae)	–50%
9	2 mile (Ae); 2 × 1200 m/3 min rest	–56%
10	3 mile (Ae)	–62%
11	REST (No Running)	
12	2 mile (Ae); 2 × 800 m/3 min rest	–62%
13	2 to 3 mile Warm-up only (Ae)	
14	°°°10,000 meter race°°°	

performance following the taper is psychological and the result of removing the psychological stress of hard training.

Attempts to achieve a peak performance at a specific time add another dimension to the art of training. Tapering the exercise intensity during the two weeks before a marathon should produce a positive effect on performance, since it allows time for healing and recovery of the body's energy stores. Although most runners feel an urge to perform one long run a week or two before the competition, there is little justification for such action. The training gains from a 15- to 20-mile run are usually not realized for three to four weeks. Plus, the risk of injury far outweighs the conditioning effects or the psychological boost of an over-distance run within the last two weeks before the race.

Runners ask how the frequency and length of tapering or reduced training periods will affect their conditioning. Swimming coaches have reported no loss in performance or general conditioning when their swimmers trained at 50% of their normal yardages for up to seven weeks. In some cases, swimmers who have been on reduced training regimens for nearly two months have set world records. Once the athlete has trained vigorously for a period of several months, much less training is needed to sustain that level of conditioning. In other words, you may have to train hard to achieve maximal physiological adaptations, but it may take much less training to keep that level of fitness.

For some unknown reason, tapering for peak performance seems to work effectively only a few times in a yearlong cycle of training. Inevitably, the peak performance will be lost, but can be repeated again after a period of basic, non-competitive training and relief from the psychological stress of competition.

STRATEGIES OF RACING

The tactics of competition are more a matter of artistry than science. Nevertheless, there are several points that may aid the runner in designing a competitive "battle plan."

First, the runner should remember that the primary source of energy during the early stage of a race will be the glycogen stored in the muscles. If the pace is unusually fast in the first few minutes, the quantity of glycogen used will be markedly greater and the muscles' stores will be seriously depleted. At the same time, the by-products of rapid glycogen breakdown may result in a large production of lactic acid, which increases the acidity of the muscle fibers. It is wise to run a bit slower than the desired racing pace during the first few minutes of the race, and to gradually accelerate to racing pace after the third up to the fifth minute of running. Although this plan may be impractical in races shorter than 10K, it can spare a sizeable amount of glycogen in the longer events. Proper pacing can minimize the threat of glycogen depletion and lessen the chance of premature exhaustion.

There seems to be little agreement among runners about the proper way to pace a race. Most runners have preconceived ideas or past successes with a variety of pacing patterns. It has been suggested that the maximum speed that can be maintained during a race depends on the muscles' capacity to generate energy and the runner's efficient use of that energy. Since the energy requirements increase dramatically with even slight acceleration, most physiologists advocate an even or steady pace during distance running.

Studies in the 1950s examined the effects of variable pace on the oxygen requirements and blood lactates of four well-conditioned subjects during exhaustive treadmill runs. The subjects were tested at three pace patterns: (1) constant, (2) slow to fast, and (3) fast to slow. The runners became exhausted in 3min:37s while running 1,245 meters at a constant speed of 13.9 miles per hour (4min:19s per mile). However, when they ran the first 2min:37s at 13.5 miles per hour and the last minute at 14.9 miles per hour, the subjects were able to cover the same distance in the same total time with a lower oxygen requirement and less blood lactate accumulation. When the runners ran the first 2min:37s at 14.9 miles per hour and the last minute at 13.5 miles per hour, they consumed more oxygen and had more blood lactate than when they ran at the constant speed of 13.9 miles per hour. The reader should note that these results may be specific to races of relatively short duration.

A study of heart rate responses to various pace patterns during the running of a mile revealed that the slow-fast pattern required less overall energy than the other pace patterns did. However, the fast-slow pace pattern was identified as the pattern that produced the fastest one-mile times.

In the 1970s another study was conducted on the energy required to run a 4min:37s mile, which was simulated on a treadmill. A steady paced run consisted of a constant time of 69.25 seconds for each 440 yards throughout the trial. The fast-slow-fast run involved consecutive 440 yard times of 64, 73, 73, and 67 seconds. The slow-fast pace required the subjects to run each 440-yard segment of the mile run in 71, 71, 67.5, and 67.5 seconds. The researchers concluded that when the pace varied, a significantly higher oxygen debt was incurred and that the steady-pace plan was the most efficient means of utilizing energy reserves. The best physiological plan for accomplishing the fastest time in middle distance running was a steady-pace strategy.

Additional support for steady pace effort had been offered by physiologists at Ohio State University in the 1970s. They studied the mechanical efficiency of exercise with the following distribution of effort: steady, light-heavy, and heavy-light. Their findings indicated that steady pace was significantly more efficient with regard to oxygen uptake (i.e., aerobic energy used). But the best racing plan still seems debatable, since other studies have found no detrimental effects of varying the pace during a 1,320-yard run. Clearly, experts don't seem to agree on the optimal pace for distance running. The steady-pace plan, however, seems to hold the greatest scientific support.

In selecting the best running speed for any given distance race, the runner should remember that running pace is limited by his/her capacity to consume oxygen and to tolerate fatigue. A series of investigations concerning the energy expenditure during various distance races has demonstrated a close relationship between the distance of the race and the $\%\dot{V}o_2max$ used by the runner. Runners competing in the two-mile, for example, were found to consume oxygen at a level equal to their maximal capacity (100% $\%\dot{V}o_2max$), whereas runners competing in six-mile and marathon races used 88 to 94% and 68 to 75% $\%\dot{V}o_2max$, respectively. This fractional use of the aerobic capacity is responsible for a runner's sensations of effort and ultimately dictates his or her running pace.

Although little attention has been given to the biomechanical skills of distance running, this topic has been discussed in some detail elsewhere (see: Slocum, D. B. and W. Bowerman). There is evidence to support the tactic of running in the aerodynamic shadow or draft of one's competition, since the energy needed to overcome the resistance of air increases exponentially with running velocity or headwind resistance. To gain full advantage of this technique, it is best to permit two or three runners to "break the way," setting up a draft for you to run in. However, in order to benefit from this technique, you need to stay close behind the other runners, perhaps within a meter of them.

During the latter stage of a race, care should be taken to reserve one's finishing sprint until the final 150 to 200 meters. Although it may seem tactically wise to increase the pace to break free of a competitor, runners should feel as though they still have some energy in reserve. Such timing is supported by knowledge about the muscle's energy supply of CP and ATP (see Chapter 2). These high-energy compounds permit the explosive energy needed for an all-out sprint. During the final dash, CP decreases rapidly, followed by a fall in muscle ATP levels. The trick is to begin the final sprint as early as possible without running out of energy short of the finish. If the runner's pace has been relatively steady, then the muscle energy stores should be sufficient to sustain a sprint lasting roughly 20 to 30 seconds.

RECOVERY FROM COMPETITION

Though recovery from some races is no more distressful than the aftermath of a typical training run, most runners have experienced the painful hours and days that follow an all-out effort of a marathon. Despite variations in the degree of discomfort after competition or other long runs, there are a number of specific physiological and anatomical changes that can be blamed for the painful side effects.

In 1977, exercise physiologists studied the biochemical changes in the blood of six runners during a marathon race and for three days afterward. Probably the most interesting finding of this study was the persistently elevated epinephrine (adrenaline) levels in the days following the race. This hormone is normally secreted by the adrenal glands in response to both physical and emotional stress, and it exhibits a strong influence on energy production and the excitability of the nervous system. Like other hormones, such as glucagon, norepinephrine, and cortisol, the amount of epinephrine is dramatically increased during the marathon. While these other hormones returned to normal levels within 24 hours after the race, epinephrine remained elevated for 24 to 48 hours after the competition (Figure 7-6). Though this persistence of an elevated epinephrine level seems to have little effect on the body's use of fuels during the recovery period, it may be responsible for the heightened psychological state that is known to persist for 24 to 48 hours after the marathon. Marathoners commonly have great difficulty sleeping for one or two nights after the marathon, which may reflect the effect of epinephrine on the central nervous system.

As noted earlier, muscle glycogen is used as a primary fuel during the early stages of the race. Fortunately, not every cell runs out of glycogen at the same time. Typically, there are always some cells that have not been extensively used. Fatigue comes in stages with the selective glycogen exhaustion of different groups of muscle fibers. The fibers that were easily recruited by the nervous system in the early part of the race no longer respond to signals from the nerves. Trying to maintain the pace, the runner concentrates harder in an attempt to activate the muscle fibers that were somewhat dormant in the first stages of the run. The smooth, comfortable pace that allowed the runner to enjoy the scenery

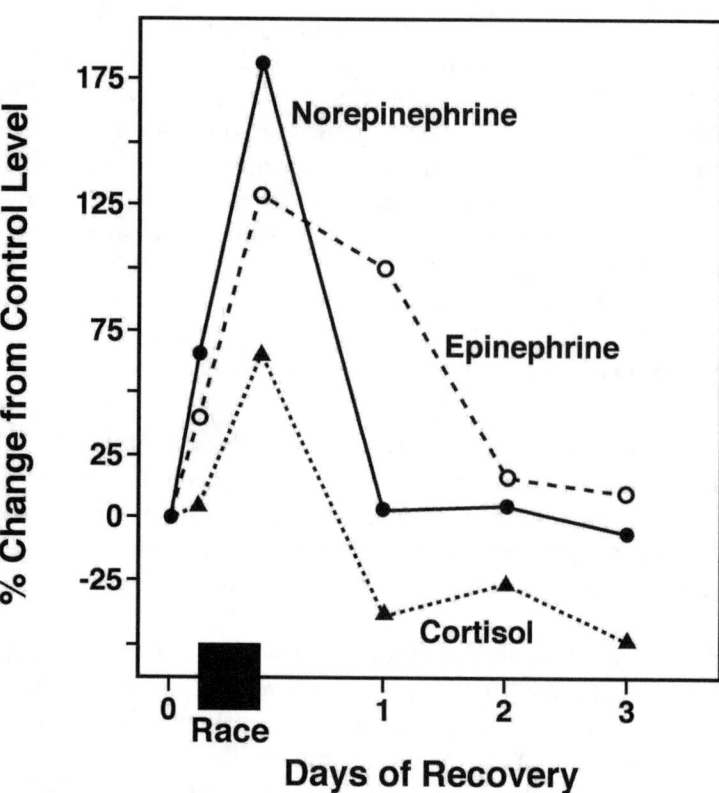

in the early stage of the race is gradually replaced by a strained effort that occupies the runner's entire concentration. The observable changes that occur in the runner's form over the final miles of a marathon can be attributed to an emptying of the muscle cells' glycogen. Unfortunately, recovery of the energy reserves necessary to resume normal running does not come quickly.

Admittedly, one of the most interesting studies we have conducted with distance runners involved taking biopsies from the calf muscles of ten competitors before and soon after the finish of the Athens (Ohio) Marathon. The specific goal of this study was to determine the rate of recovery during the first week after the race. Additional muscle samples were taken one, three, five, and seven days following the marathon. Portions of the muscle specimens were analyzed for glycogen content, and a small part of each biopsy was studied under an electron microscope to determine if the marathon had caused any structural damage.

Four of the 10 men placed in the top 13 places (1st, 2nd, 4th, and 13th) out of a field of 350 runners. Although all the runners were exhausted by the race, two of the slower runners, whose times were 3h:8min and 3h:17min, were the most devastated by their efforts. Both men lay collapsed and unwilling to move for nearly two hours after the race, and experienced severe muscle soreness for the next six to 7 days. Though all of the runners started the race with very large amounts of muscle glycogen of 196 mmol/kg muscle (normal values for untrained men 80-100 mmol/kg), at the finish they all had less than 25 mmol/kg muscle. The two most exhausted runners had less than 8 mmol/kg of muscle.

The Recovery of Muscle Glycogen

Our research has taught us that the fastest way to recover the used muscle glycogen is to eat extremely large quantities of carbohydrates like bread and pasta, much as you might do prior to a marathon. The day following the marathon our subjects ate 400 grams of carbohydrate, nearly three times the normal daily carbohydrate intake. Despite this large carbohydrate intake, the runners' muscle glycogen levels averaged only 79 mmol/kg muscle 24 hours after the race, far below their starting level. During the week that followed the race, the men ate roughly 450 grams of carbohydrate each day. Despite this rich carbohydrate diet, several of the runners did not return to their pre-race glycogen levels a week after the race.

Since some authorities have suggested that moderate exercise in the week after a marathon might accelerate recovery, we divided the 10 runners into two groups. One group rested completely during the recovery week, while the other five men ran on a treadmill for 20 to 45 minutes per day at an easy pace. Over that period of time the muscle glycogen restoration was the same in both groups, reaching a high value of 131 mmol/kg muscle on the fifth day. Although this muscle glycogen value is well below the pre-race value, it is a level we often see in trained runners. In addition to the glycogen value similarities, the groups displayed no differences in the subjective sensations of muscle soreness or general fatigue. These facts suggest that light exercise following a marathon does not expedite recovery. In otherwords, it probably doesn't make much difference whether you start running again in the days after an exhaustive race like the marathon. You will recover from the race at the same rate whether you exercise or not.

We have considered a number of possible explanations for the somewhat incomplete recovery of muscle glycogen after the marathon. At first we thought it might be a disadvantage to take in so much carbohydrate during the first 24 hours after the race. We reasoned that overloading the system with carbohydrate in such a brief time period might suppress the enzyme activity that promotes glycogen. However, more recent studies in our lab suggest that the muscle damage and subsequent inflammatory reactions that occur during distance running may attenuate the rate of muscle glycogen formation. We have observed that when muscle fibers are damaged after exercise that causes sorness, they store 40% less glycogen than undamaged muscles. At the time of the Athens Marathon study we had yet to confirm that marathon running caused any damage to the muscle.

Muscle Trauma From Running

A team of specialists at Ohio University, headed by Robert Hikida, examined small pieces of the muscles under an electron microscope. As noted earlier in this chapter, the findings were quite surprising. In nearly all samples studied, including those taken before the race, there was evidence of ruptured fibers and inflammation within the muscle (Figures 7-1, 7-2a, and 7-2b). Many of the substances normally confined to the inside of the cells were found outside the fibers in the fluids that bathe the muscle cells. Even red and white blood cells were found outside the blood vessels. Occasionally the observers noted derangements in the contractile filaments (Figures 7-2a and 7-2b). Because the abnormalities were found in the pre-marathon samples and persisted for a week after the race, it seems that these changes were caused by the intensity of both training and racing. It even appears that the inflammatory reaction that accompanies such running may be a major cause for the post-exercise symptoms of muscle soreness.

Why does this trauma occur during an event like the marathon? Does it also happen during other endurance events like cycling and swimming? Studies at the University of Limburg in The Netherlands revealed that cyclists and swimmers do not experience the muscle fiber damage and soreness observed in runners. So, there must be something special about running that other forms of exercise do not contain.

That "something" is likely due to the eccentric contractions that occur during running. Concentric contractions normally shorten the muscle in the process of developing force, while eccentric contractions involve lengthening the muscle at the same time it is attempting to shorten. Bending the elbow and shortening the biceps muscle, for example, involves concentric contractions, but following this movement with a slow extension, lowering the weight, will develop additional tension as the biceps muscle is stretched while attempting to slowly lower the weight. It is a bit like stretching a rubberband too far. It will produce tension as you pull on it, but eventually it will break. In running, the concentric forces generated by the leg muscles are used to drive the body forward, while the eccentric contractions of the thigh muscles prevent the knee and hip from yielding to the pull of gravity when the heel strikes the ground.

In downhill running, the tension developed in the leg muscles to resist gravity is enormous. The muscles are attempting to shorten but are literally pulled apart. Consequently, the fiber membranes and connective tissues are physically stretched beyond their limits. The next obvious questions are: Is this muscle damage permanent? Does it ultimately impair performance? There is no evidence that these disruptions in the muscle cell membranes and microcirculation cause any permanent damage. Studies with both humans and small animals have shown that the muscle is easily capable of repairing itself. In rats it has even been shown that the muscle will reconstructed itself after being excised (removed), minced, and replaced in the original muscle compartment. Within about 30 days, a competent whole muscle, complete with tendon and nerve connections, will be regenerated. The muscle makes a few modifications during such regeneration, becoming more fibrous with added connective tissue to make it more tolerant of future sorts of damage and/or eccentric stresses. It also seems that the more a person performs eccentric exercise, the less soreness and muscle trauma they experience.

One of the after effects of a long exhaustive run is the loss of muscle strength and power, which may persist for several days. During the Athens Marathon study we compared the effects of complete rest and mild exercise on the rate of strength recovery during seven days after a marathon. Both the rest-recovery and exercise-recovery groups regained some of their loss of muscle function during the first three days of recovery. Though both groups continued to regain leg strength, five days after the marathon the men who had rested completely showed a greater recovery of both leg extension strength and work capacity (Figure 7-7). While the work capacity of the leg muscles may return to normal with adequate rest, muscle strength remained depressed even after seven days of rest. Again, these and other findings raise doubts about the value of exercise during the days following an exhaustive event like the marathon.

Certainly there are other physiological and psychological aspects of recovery from long-distance running that have not been covered here. Current evidence, however, makes it clear that recovery from events like the marathon involve nutrition recovery and the healing of damaged tissues. Though some aspects of recovery may be accomplished within a few hours, others may require a month or more.

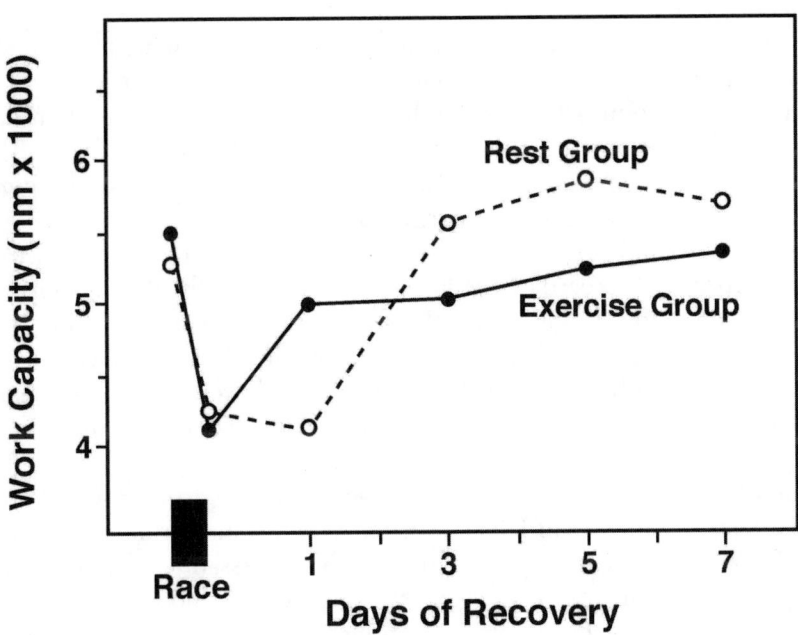

Figure 7-7. Changes in leg extension work capacity as a result of the marathon and during recovery. The rest group did no running for seven days after the marathon, whereas the exercise group ran 20 to 45 min per day at 50 to 60% VO_2max during the recovery week. Note the difference between the rate of recovery of the two groups.

DETRAINING: USE IT OR LOSE IT

Most athletes agree that it is bad enough to suffer the pain of an injury, but it is even worse when the condition forces them to stop training. Aside from the psychological trauma of such inactivity, runners fear most that all they have gained through hard training will be lost after a few days or weeks without running. The discussion on tapering made it clear that a few days of rest or a reduction in training will enhance performance, not diminish it. Runners realize, however, that at some point a reduction in training or inactivity will impact their conditioning and performance.

Apparently, it takes much less daily exercise to sustain the aerobic benefits of endurance training than it does initially to increase one's aerobic capacity. Unfortunately, the fitness gained from miles and miles of running are quickly lost when the runner stops all training. With the cessation of training, improvements in $\dot{V}O_2$max, maximal cardiac output, skeletal muscle capillarization, and the aerobic capacity of the leg muscles vanish at varied rates. If for some reason the endurance athlete is unable to train for just one week, the muscles' aerobic capacity may decline by 10 to 50%. This finding is supported by observations that the activities of the mitochondrial enzymes are markedly reduced with the cessation of exercise training. Some physiologists have shown that the enzymes may begin to decline within just 48 hours if muscles are not exercised. After an additional week of inactivity, the muscles' aerobic capacity remains depressed, though trained muscles still have far more endurance than untrained muscles. Despite these changes at the muscle level, running performance may show only small decrements in the first week or two of inactivity.

Another important change that takes place with detraining is a decrease in the number of capillaries that surround each muscle fiber that deliver oxygen and nutrients to the muscle cells. Studies have shown that the number of capillaries around each muscle fiber decreases by 10 to 20% within five to 12 days after the last training session. As a result, the delivery of oxygen to these muscle cells and their ability to produce energy may be impaired.

During the same period of detraining, significant changes take place in the central portion of the cardiovascular system. Specifically, the capacity of the heart to pump blood during maximal effort begins to decrease within the first five to 12 days of inactivity. The combination of a lower maximal cardiac output and a smaller blood flow around the muscle fibers lessens the transport of oxygen to the runner's muscle fibers and slows the removal of waste materials from the working muscles.

One of these waste products is lactic acid, the result of muscular effort to produce energy without sufficient oxygen. A well-trained runner accumulates very little blood lactate during long runs. With the cessation of training and the subsequent weakening of the oxygen transport system, blood lactate levels are substantially higher during aerobic-anaerobic running. Figure 7-8 demonstrates

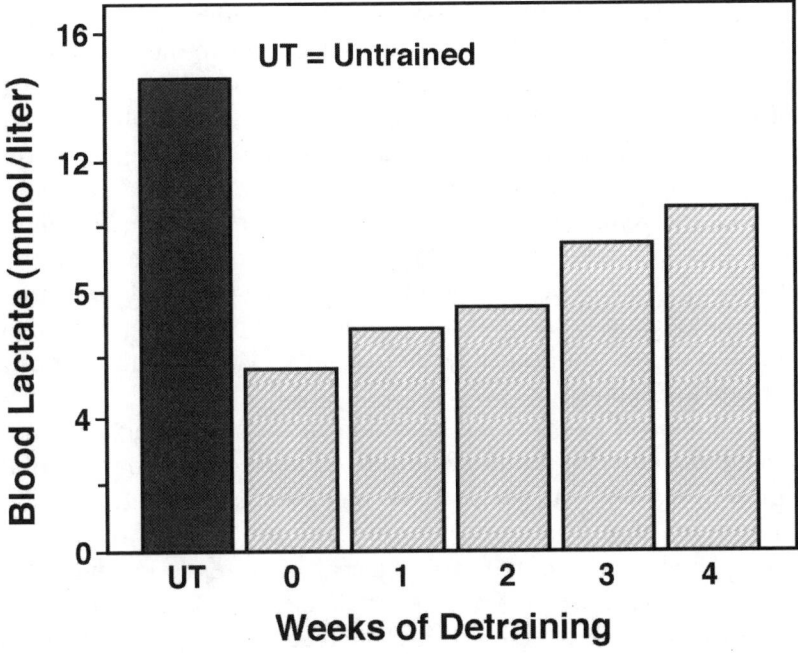

Figure 7-8. Effects of training and detraining on blood lactate concentration after a treadmill run at a predetermined pace of 6-minutes per mile.

the changes in blood lactate concentration for a runner who performed a six-minute mile when he was untrained, after five months of training, and at weekly intervals during a period of inactivity. Note that by the fourth week of detraining, blood lactate is well on its way to reaching the untrained level. We estimate that with six to 8 weeks of detraining the runner will have lost all of the endurance advantage gained from the five months of training.

All physiological changes associated with the muscles' ability to produce energy do not decline at the same rate when the runner stops training. The real question is: "How quickly will performance be affected after the runner stops training?" In general, there is no loss for five to 7 days. As a matter of fact, running performance may even be improved after two to 5 days of inactivity. As noted earlier, such rest periods allow the muscles and nervous system to recover and rebuild from the stress of training and provide the runner with improved energy reserves and tolerance of endurance exercise.

Taking a few days of rest before a major competition to enhance one's muscle glycogen stores is a common practice among most runners. Prior training plays a key role in this process of muscle glycogen storage. Runners who are well-trained, rested, and properly fed have 50 to 100% more muscle glycogen than untrained individuals. With detraining, this fuel advantage is gradually lost, and by the fourth week of inactivity, muscle glycogen levels in an idle athlete may be no better than those in an untrained individual. Such a change would be noticed by the runner as an inability to do a long run or to train hard on two or more consecutive days, though he or she might be able to do one run and feel fine.

Although most runners train year-round, injuries often demand a few weeks or months of inactivity. Recently, some physiologists have suggested that a substitute form of exercise might delay the loss of muscle conditioning. Though it is true that riding a bike and swimming may continue to stimulate the heart and respiratory muscles, such activities are not specific to running. Consequently, those special changes that take place in and around the runner's muscles are lost, as if the runner were doing no exercise at all. Activities that simulate the action of running, however, may delay this loss of muscle conditioning. Performing a running action in shallow or deep water may provide sufficient stress to stimulate energy production in some of the muscles used in running, thereby maintaining these systems. Unfortunately, there is no activity that can serve as a perfect substitute for running.

Though it appears that the physiological gains from training are short-lived in detraining, the rate of retraining seems to be affected by the status of conditioning prior to the lapse. A classical study on detraining and retraining demonstrated an average 26% decrease in $\dot{V}O_2$max levels in a group of runners after 20 days of complete bed rest. In the two subjects who were most active before the bed rest period, one to two months of retraining were needed to regain their aerobic capacities. The least active subjects in that study improved their $\dot{V}O_2$max values rapidly after the period of bed rest, returning to the initial levels with only 10 to 15 days of training. As illustrated in Figure 7-9, the difference in the rate of retraining the $\dot{V}O_2$max level may be related to the initial fitness of the subjects. Those individuals with the highest level of fitness prior to complete bed rest appear to suffer the greatest decrements in $\dot{V}O_2$max and the slowest recovery during retraining.

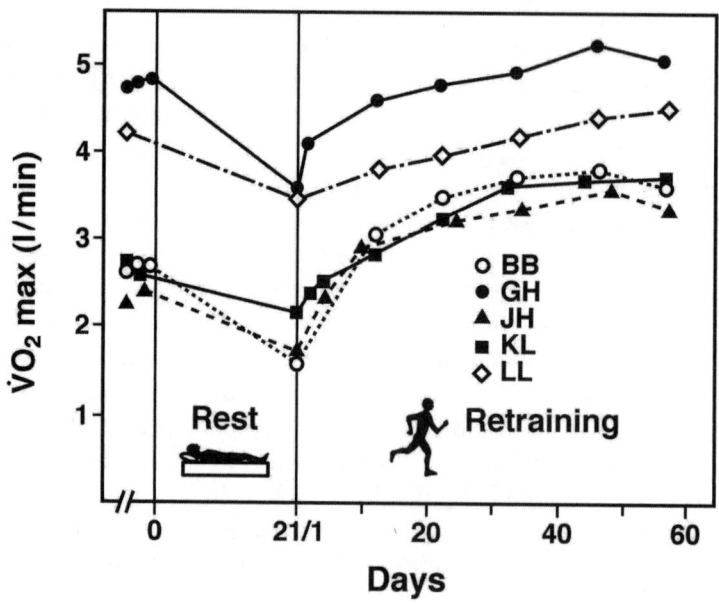

Figure 7-9. *Maximal oxygen uptake in five men who were subjected to bed rest for 20 days and thereafter underwent a physical conditioning program for 55 days. Subjects GH and LL were physically active prior to the start of the study, whereas subjects BB, JH, and KL were sedentary before the study.*

178

RUNNING: THE ATHLETE WITHIN

After a layoff of more than two weeks, a runner should not expect an immediate return to his or her original state of fitness. Because of the weakened state, the runner who is trying to retrain is quite susceptible to becoming chronically fatigued and glycogen depleted. Consequently, care must be taken to initiate the training at a low intensity and to progress back to the pre-layoff level over a two- to four-week period.

The physiological gains of training are short-lived when regular activity ceases. Though moderate amounts of running can maintain performance levels for many weeks, total inactivity can mean a loss of all training benefits within a few months. Our laboratory tests have shown that even the most gifted distance runners are indistinguishable from the sedentary individual after 6 to 12 months of inactivity. To accommodate the stress of running competition, the body tissues must constantly be reminded of the physiological and biochemical demands of maximal effort. Without such reinforcement, the benefits of training are lost.

FINER POINTS OF TRAINING

The preceding discussion provides a number of general and specific principles that are important for runners to achieve their best performances. Certainly, our limited knowledge of individual variations in response to training precludes the development of a single racing strategy that will work equally well for all runners. Nevertheless, previous research offers some guidelines that are essential if the runner hopes to attain a peak in performance.

1. Enough is enough. A gradual progression in training stress enhances the muscles' capacity to generate energy and remove the by-products of intense exercise. Improvements in fitness result from a balance between exercise and rest. Excessive training stress or inadequate recovery time or both cause a breakdown in adaptation and a loss in conditioning. The secret of a good training program is to be able to judge how much and what type of training will produce the greatest amount of improvement in conditioning. Once an athlete is overtrained, a period of reduced training or complete rest may be necessary to regain an optimal level of performance. Reductions in the training load are also essential for maximal speed and stamina. Tapering for one to two weeks before a major competition allows time for recovery from heavy training and a reprieve from the psychological demands of exhaustive exercise. Once trained, the runner can reduce his or her training for several weeks without a measurable loss in the quality of performance. While a few days of rest may actually improve a runner's performance, several weeks of complete inactivity will lead to a rapid loss in conditioning and a deterioration in performance. Detraining for more than six to 8 weeks will lower the runner's endurance capacity to that of a sedentary individual. Retraining the runner after such a layoff requires a slow and easy start to prevent overstress.

2. Diet and rest. The keys to maximal glycogen loading are: (1) to reduce the intensity and duration of your training runs to minimize the daily burn-off of both muscle and liver glycogen stores and (2) to increase the percentage of carbohydrates in your diet. There is no reason to use a high-fat protein diet or a depletion run to stimulate extra glycogen storage. The endurance-trained muscle needs only a few days of rest and a rich carbohydrate diet to allow for maximal glycogen loading.

On the day of the race, the runner should eat a light carbohydrate meal three to 4 hours before the competition to allow for complete digestion. Substances that are hard to digest, like meat and fatty foods, should be excluded. The idea is to have as little as possible in the stomach when the race starts. In three to 4 hours even a stack of pancakes will generally be emptied into the intestine, but meat can be found in the stomach ten to 12 hours after a meal.

3. Warm-up. Some experts suggest warming up for a distance race to increase muscle temperature, prevent muscle and tendon injuries, to bring on "second wind" sooner, and to rehearse the pace and relaxation which will be required during the actual competition. Measurements of rectal temperature before and after a 10,000-meter race in hot weather demonstrate that warming up may not be wise in the heat. Studies have shown that warming up raises the internal body temperature by 1.5°F above the resting level, causing runners to risk over-heating during the race.

4. Pacing. In light of the body's limited supply of fuel and its restricted capacity to generate energy, running efficiency and pace are critical to overall performance. Although an evenly paced race strategy appears to be the best plan, the speed or rate of energy expenditure must be based on the runner's physiological limits and the environmental heat stress. Hot weather running takes a costly toll on performance and exposes the runner to the threat of heat injury. Unfortunately, many runners attempt to run at their fastest tolerable speeds, regardless of the environmental temperature.

Another common mistake in pacing comes when runners think they can run a bit faster during the early stages of the race to gain a few minutes' or seconds' advantage that might compensate for the fatigue-induced slowdown near the finish. My running partners, who hope to average eight minutes per mile for the marathon, invariably run the first 10 miles at 7min:45s, thereby gaining a 2min:30s lead on their desired overall time. Unfortunately, this slightly faster pace costs them a great deal more muscle glycogen, exhausting their fuel supplies at 18 to 22 miles, instead of at the finish. Consequently, the seconds gained in the early stage of the race are replaced by many minutes of slow running and walking. It is surprising that they cannot understand why they "hit the wall." It is simply a matter of poor pacing and an inefficient use of their energy reserves.

5. Post-race recovery. The rate of recovery from an exhaustive competition depends, to a large degree, on the amount of muscle trauma and glycogen depletion experienced during the race. It seems that a combination of rest and a carbohydrate-rich diet offers the best plan for recovery. If the runner experiences severe muscle soreness or tenderness under the pressure of palpation, there is little value in training until these symptoms have disappeared. Returning to training too soon will only delay recovery and increase the risk of overtraining. Despite both rest and carbohydrates, full recovery from an extremely exhaustive run may be relatively slow, precluding a quick return to further racing.

CLASSIC AND SUGGESTED READINGS

Armstrong, L. E., W. M. Sherman and D. L. Costill. Muscle soreness following exhaustive long distance running. *Track Field Quart. Rev.,* 82:47–51, 1982.

Brynteson, P. and W. E. Sinning. The effects of training frequencies on the retention of cardiovascular fitness. *Med. Sci. Sports,* 5:29–33, 1973.

Carlson, B. M. An investigation into a method for the stimulation of regeneration of skeletal muscle. *Anat. Rec.,* 157:225, 1967.

Chi, M. M.Y., C. S. Hitz, E. F. Coyle, W. H. Martin, J. L. Ivy, P. M. Nemeth, J. O. Holloszy and 0. H. Lowry. Effects of detraining on enzymes of energy metabolism in individuals human muscle fiber. *Am. J. Physiol.,* 224:C276–C287, 1983.

Costill, D. L. Metabolic responses during distance running. *J. Appl. Physiol.,* 28:251.

Costill, D. L., D. S. King, R. Thomas and M. Hargreaves. Effects of reduced training on muscular power in swimmers. *Physician & Sportsmed.,*13:94–101, 1985.

Costill, D. L., W. J. Fink, M. Hargreaves, D. S. King, R. Thomas and R. Fielding. Metabolic characteristics of skeletal muscle during detraining from competitive swimming. *Med. Sci. Sports Exer.,* 17:339–343, 1985.

Coyle, E. F., W. H. Martin and J. O. Holloszy. Cardiovascular and metabolic rates of detraining. *Med. Sci. Sports Exer.,* 15:158, 1983.

Forsburg, A., P. Tesch and J. Karlsson. Effect of prolonged exercise on muscle strength performance. *Biomechanics VI-A,* 6:62–67, 1979.

Friden, J. Muscle soreness after exercise: Implications of morphological changes. *Int. J. Sports Med.,* 5:57–66, 1984.

Hagerman, F. C., R. S. Hikida, R. S. Staron, W. M. Sherman and D. L. Costill. Muscle damage in marathon runners. *Physician and Sportsmed.,* 12:39–48, 1984.

Hickson, R. C., J. M. Hagbert, A. A. Ehsani and 1. O. Holloszy. Time course of the increase in V_{O_2}max in response to training. *Fed. Proc.,* 37:633, 1978.

Hickson, R. C., J. C. Kanakis, A. M. Moore and S. Rich. Effects of frequency of training, reduced training and retraining on aerobic power and left ventricular responses. *Med. Sci. Sports Exercise,* 13:93, 1981.

Hikida, R. S., R. S. Staron, F. C. Hagerman, W. M. Sherman and D. L. Costill. Muscle fiber necrosis associated with human marathon runners. *J. Neuro. Sci.,* 59:185–203, 1983.

Houmard, J.A., B.K. Scott, C.L. Justice, and T.C. Chenier. The effects of taper on performance in distance runners. *Med. Sci. Sports Exerc.,* 26: 624–631, 1994.

Houmard, J.A., D.L. Costill, J.B. Mitchell, S.H. Park, R.C. Hickner, and J.N. Roemmich. Reduced training maintains perforomance in distance runners. *Int. J. Sports Med.* 11:46–52, 1990.

Houston, M. E., H. Bentzen and H. Larsen. Interrelationships between skeletal muscle adaptations and performance as studied by detraining and retraining. *Acta Physiol. Scand.*, 105:163–170, 1979.

Kanakis, C., A. Coehlo and R. C. Hickson. Left ventricular responses to strenuous endurance training and reduced training frequencies. *J. Cardiac Rehab.*, 2:141–146, 1982.

Maglischo, E. W. *Swimming Faster*, 368–375. Palo Alto: Mayfield Publishing Co., 1982.

Robinson, S. Influence of fatigue on the efficiency of men during exhaustive runs. *J. Appl. Physiol.*, 12:197–201, 1958.

Saltin, B., G. Blomquist, J. H. Mitchell, J. R. L. Johnson, K. Wildenthal and C. B. Chapman. Response to exercise after bedrest and after training. *Circulation*, (Suppl.) 7:1968.

Selye, H. *The Stress of Life*, 324. New York: McGraw-Hill, 1956.

Sherman, W. M., D. L. Costill, W. J. Fink, F. C. Hagerman, L. E. Armstrong and T. F. Murray. Effect of a 42.2-km footrace and subsequent rest or exercise on muscle glycogen and enzymes. *J. Appl. Physiol.*, 55:1219–1224, 1983.

Sherman, W. M., L. E. Armstrong, T. M. Murray, F. C. Hagerman, D. L. Costill, R. C. Staron and J. L. Ivy. Effect of a 42.2-km footrace and subsequent rest or exercise on muscular strength and work capacity. *J. Appl. Physiol.*, 57:1668–1673, 1984.

Index

C

caffeine, fat use promotion, 59
calcium, human sweat component, 64
capillaries, muscle training increase, 75–76
carbohydrate (glycogen)
    blood glucose contribution, 52
    dietary down-sides, 55
    dietary effects on muscle glycogen, 53–55
    during distance competition, 60–61
    liver glycogen replenishment, 57
    muscle fuel, 34–39, 51–52
    pre-race intake timing, 58
    sports drinks, 66, 67
    types, 56
carbon dioxide, running by-product, 42
cardiac output, defined, 16
cardiovascular system
    dehydration impact, 63–64
    distance running responses, 39–41
    maximal heart rate, 81–82
    older runners, 135–140
    pregnancy demands, 122–123
    respirations, 41–42
    training adaptations, 81–82
Castagnola, Lou, 24
cereal, pre-race food, 58
chloride, blood water content responsibility, 64
cholesterol, high density lipoprotein cholesterol (HDLC), 23
Clayton, Derek, 5, 15, 17, 28, 30, 136–137
coffee, international competition restrictions, 59
cold fluids
    body cooling enhancement, 65
    stomach emptying rates, 65–66
cold weather, training guidelines, 99–100, 103
cold/hot weather, training plan factor, 103
competition, recovery, 171–175
conditioning, training plan element, 91–92
Corbitt, Ted, 28–29
CPK (creatine phosphokinase), overtraining, 159
cramps
    heat effect, 47–48
    stomach distress caused by fluid intake, 65
cyclists, muscle glycogen depletion, 36

D

dehydration
    aldosterone release, 65
    cardiovascular system impact, 63–64
    distance runner's fluid loss rate, 63
DeMar, Clarence, 18–19
detraining, performance, 176–179
diets
    exercise importance, 71–72
    fluids, 63–68
    glycogen loading, 56–58
    minerals, 71
    pre-race foods, 58–59
    runner's Recommended Daily Allowance (RDA), 61–63
    sports drinks, 66
    supplements, 68–71
    vitamins, 68–71
distance runners
    10k training plan, 92–94
    aerodynamic shadow (drafting), 34
    breathing rates, 41–42
    by-products, 42–44
    carbohydrate feedings during race, 60–61
    cardiovascular system responses, 39–41
    dehydration avoidance, 63
    eating habits, 61–63
    efficiency examination, 28–30
    energy needs, 27–28
    enlarged left ventricles, 17
    exhaustion factors, 12
    fat burning importance, 13
    female, 106–128
    fluid intake during race, 67–68
    four-week "beginner" training plan, 92
    heat affects, 45–48
    hematocrit (red blood cells), 22–23
    hyponatremia risks, 66
    marathon training plan, 94–96
    maximal heart rate (%HR max) measurement, 20–21
    maximal oxygen uptake ($\dot{V}O_2max$), 13–16
    maximum breathing capacity (MBC) measurement, 21
    muscle groups, 6–11
    overtraining, 162
    oxygen consumption measurement study, 33
    oxygen delivery limits, 30–34
    physiques, 2–6
    single fiber function, 150–152
    strength training, 96–97
    strength/speed testing, 24

Human Performance Laboratory, older runner physical traits, 132–141
HV (heart volume), gender comparisons, 116
hypoglycemia
    blood changes during long runs, 44
    risk lessening, 52
hyponatremia, defined, 66
hypotonic, defined, 64

I

identical twins, muscle fiber type, 10
injuries
    heat exhaustion, 47–48
    heat stroke, 47
    muscle cramping, 47–48
International Olympic Committee, coffee/tea restrictions, 59
interval training
    aerobic intervals, 86–87
    aerobic-anaerobic intervals, 87–89
    anerobic, 90
    race pace, 87–89
iron, female runner supplement, 118

J

joints, older runner considerations, 152–153
juice, pre-race food, 58

K

Khannouchi, Khalid, 131
kidneys
    electrolyte management, 65
    water per hour loss rate, 64

L

lactate (lactic acid)
    endurance level indicator, 31
    running by-product, 42
lateral meniscus injuries, older runners, 152
LDH (lactase dehydrogen), overtraining, 159
leg strength, male/female comparisons, 119
legs, muscle fiber types, 11
lipids (fats), energy source, 38–39
lipoproteins, 23
liver, fuel storage, 34
liver glucose, hypoglycemia risk lessening, 52
liver glycogen
    breakdown, 38
    monitoring techniques, 57–58

rapid decrease w/carbohydrate deprivation, 57
low blood sodium (hyponatremia), 66
lungs
    breathing rates, 41–42
    maximum breathing capacity (MBC) measurement, 21
    oxygen delivery training, 79–80
    oxygen/carbon dioxide mixture, 41
    pregnancy demands, 123
    respirations, 41–42
    tidal volume, 123
    vital capacity, 21, 139

M

Maglischo, Ernie (swimming coach), 166
magnesium, human sweat component, 64
males
    body fat percentages, 2–3
    maximal oxygen uptake ($\dot{V}O_2max$), 14
    performance decline w/age, 131
    performance/gender factors, 106–108
marathon runners
    fiber membrane disruption, 159
    tapering training, 167
    training plan, 94–96
master athlete. See older runners
maximal breathing capacity (MBC)
    described, 21
    pregnancy effect, 123
maximal heart rate (%HR max)
    cardiovascular system, 81–82
    described, 20–21
    older runners, 139–140
maximal oxygen uptake ($\dot{V}O_2max$)
    described, 13–16
    gender comparisons, 116–118
    older runners, 135–138
    training gain, 82
MBC (maximum breathing capacity)
    described, 21
    pregnancy effect, 123
McDonagh, Jim, 28–29
medial meniscus injuries, older runners, 152
menstruation, bone mineral densities (BMD), 111–113
Metropolitan Life Insurance, height/weight charts, 4
minerals, 71
mitochondria, aerobic energy production (AEP), 76–77

mitochondria, ATP production, 11–12
muscle composition, female runners, 113–114
muscle fibers
    distance runner age changes, 147–148
    elite distance runner's single fiber function, 150–152
    older runner examination, 148–150
    older runner's composition, 145–147
    succinate dehydrogenase (SDH) marker, 148
muscle fuels
    adenosine triphosphate (ATP) storage, 51
    blood glucose, 52
    carbohydrates, 51–56, 60–61
    fats as energy source, 52
    female runner delivery systems, 114–116
    fluids, 63–68
    free fatty acids (FFA), 58–59
    glycogen refueling, 52
    liver glucose, 52, 57
    minerals, 71
    pre-competition glycogen loading, 56–58
    pregnancy alterations, 124
    pregnancy considerations, 125
    pre-race foods, 58–59
    Recommended Daily Allowance (RDA), 61–63
    sports drinks, 66
    supplements during pregnancy, 125
    vitamins, 68–71
muscle glycogen, recovery after marathon, 173
muscle mass
    distance runners, 2
    older runner retention methods, 144–145
    older runners, 134
    weight loss considerations, 3
muscle strength, age-related decline, 142–144
muscles
    adenosine triphosphate (ATP) sources, 11–12
    biopsy procedure, 6–8
    blood changes during long runs, 44–45
    cramping, 47–48
    delivery systems, 22–24
    fast-twitch (type IIa/IIb) fiber, 8–11
    fat burning importance, 13
    female runner strength/speed factors, 119–121
    fiber types, 6–11
    fuel storage, 34–39

gastro-cnemius, 11
gastrocnemius, 12
genetic effect on fiber type, 6, 10
glycogen depletion measurement, 77–78
heat exhaustion, 47–48
heat stroke, 47
maximal oxygen uptake ($\dot{V}O_2$max) measurement, 13–16
mitochondria, 11–12
myoglobin, 76
pH values, 43
selective activation, 9–10
slow-twitch (type I) fiber, 8–11
soleus, 11
sprinters versus distance runners, 6–11
terrain variation affects, 33
training transformations, 75–79
trauma from running, 174–175
myoglobin, oxygen delivery, 76

N

Nurmi, Paavo, 17
nutrition, pregnancy considerations, 125

O

OBLA (onset of blood lactate accumulation), endurance indicator, 31
older runners
    body composition, 133–135
    body fat, 134
    body weight maintenance, 133–134
    bone health, 153–154
    cardiovascular system, 135–140
    distance runner muscle changes, 147–148
    distance runner's single fiber function, 150–152
    fast-twitch fibers, 146–147
    lifestyle changes, 137
    maximal heart rate, 139–140
    maximal oxygen uptake ($\dot{V}O_2$max), 135–138
    muscle changes w/age, 142–144
    muscle fiber composition, 145–150
    muscle mass, 134, 144–145
    orthopedics, 152–153
    performance trends, 129–132
    physical traits, 132–141
    resistance-training guidelines, 144–145
    running economy, 140–141
    sarcopenia, 144

sweat loss/body weight, 64
training/muscle fiber capillary increase, 75–76
respirations, cardiovascular system, 41–42
respiratory system
altitude training, 100–102
oxygen delivery training, 79–80
pregnancy demands, 123
tidal volume, 123
rest/work balance, training plan factor, 103
Rodgers, Bill, 14–15
runners
beginning, four-week training plan, 92
body shape/composition, 2–6
body weight, 3
born versus made, 1–2
muscle groups, 6–11
running economy, master runners, 140–141

S

Salazar, Alberto, 2, 4, 14–15, 27
sarcopenia, weight training as prevention method, 144
sclerosis, older runners, 153
SCOT (serum glutamic oxaloacetic transaminase), overtraining, 159
SDH (succinate dehydrogenase), aerobic potential marker, 148
Sheehan, George, 84
Shorter, Frank, 2, 14–15, 30
Shrubb, Alfred, 85
skinfold thickness, body fat measurement method, 3
slow-twitch (type I) muscle fiber
described, 8–11
female runners, 113–114
glycogen depletion rate, 77–78
muscle glycogen depletion, 36–38
older runners, 145–147
sodium, blood water content responsibility, 64
soleus muscle, fiber types, 11
specificity, training plan factor, 103
speed training, 90
speed, female runners, 119–121
sports anemia, defined, 118
sports drinks
carbohydrate type, 56
cautions/concerns, 66
palatability, 67–68
versus water, 67

sprinters
type II (fast-twitch) muscle fiber, 8
versus distance runner's muscles, 6–11
starch, carbohydrate type, 56
stomach
drink osmolality effect, 66
fluid emptying rates, 65–66
strength, female runners, 119–121
strength training. See also weight training
distance runners, 96–97
muscle mass retention in older runners, 144–145
succinate dehydrogenase (SDH), aerobic potential marker, 148
sugars
carbohydrate type, 56
pre-race intake timing, 58
supplements
iron, 118
minerals, 71
pregnancy, 125
vitamins, 68–71
sweat
aldosterone release, 65
electrolyte concentrations, 64
filtrate of plasma, 64
hypotonic, 64

T

table sugar, carbohydrate type, 56
tapering
optimizing performance, 165–169
swimmers versus runners, 167
teas, international competition restrictions, 59
terrain, muscle stress affects, 33
thermoregulation, pregnancy concerns, 123
tidal volume, pregnancy effect, 123
tissue glycogen, carbohydrate intake, 52
toast, pre-race food, 58
tolerance, training plan element, 91
trainability, female runners, 121–122
training
10K runs, 92–94
aerobic intervals, 86–87
aerobic-anaerobic intervals, 87–89
altitude, 100–103
anaerobic interval, 90
avoid overtraining, 179
blood doping, 80–81
cardiovascular system, 81–82